Mental Fitness

Transforming Minds, A Personal Trainer's Guide

CHARLES T. ROBINSON JR.

authorHOUSE®

AuthorHouse™
1663 Liberty Drive
Bloomington, IN 47403
www.authorhouse.com
Phone: 1-800-839-8640

First published by AuthorHouse 2/7/2011

ISBN: 978-1-4520-8539-5 (sc)
ISBN: 978-1-4520-8540-1 (dj)
ISBN: 978-1-4520-8541-8 (e)

Library of Congress Control Number: 2011900457

Printed in the United States of America

To my late sister, Jessica L. Robinson

Contents

Acknowledgments

To my parents, Charles and Deborah Robinson, and to my sister Marilyn Robinson for being supportive, always having an open ear, and believing in my dreams;

Elder Gladys Henderson-Williams for giving a helping hand and sharing her vast wisdom;

Eddie and Sonya Mason for allowing me to be a part of their family, believing in the purpose God has for my life, and contributing to my dream;

Lakia Gordon for helping me get this project off the ground;

everyone else who has been a blessing to my life;

and last but definitely not least, to my Lord and Savior for blessing me to be a blessing to others.

Abbreviations

AMP   The Amplified Bible (Grand Rapids, MI: Zondervan, 1987).

KJV   King James Version

NIV   New International Version (Wheaton, IL: Tyndale House Publishers, 2005).

Preface

It was mid-January, late at night, five minutes after twelve to be exact, when I felt the compulsion to script this material. I was lying on my bed, gazing at the ceiling and praying. There I lay, fixated on the thought of how I could possibly help others achieve more, and then it struck me. A thought crossed my mind: *You always wanted to write a book. Why not turn to your passion and write a book about it?* I had found my passion in helping people think at a higher level than they normally were accustomed to doing.

The knowledge and inspiration I received for writing this book came from being a lifelong athlete and going through the process of training to be a professional athlete. During the time of training for professional athletics, I was successful in seeing the mentality of professional athletes firsthand. I trained alongside some well-known and exceptional athletes. During this stint, I also worked full-time as a personal trainer and gained valuable wisdom. I thought it was interesting that those I trained, being average people who had never played a professional sport, showed a commitment and dedication to their physical health similar to that of the professional athletes I trained alongside. Many of those I trained showed a fierce commitment to their own betterment.

I saw that in all endeavors in life, the people who get results are the ones who believe they can. Also, working as a personal trainer, I saw the correlation between physical health and mental health, physical stamina and mental stamina, physical strength and mental strength. Throughout my entire life, I have carried a fascination with understanding why people think as they do. I was intrigued by the mental qualities of people, and as a result, I brought together my interest in the mind and my love for training. I thought that as a personal trainer, I could provide a unique perspective on the training of the mind.

A personal trainer is an instructor who instructs the client on the proper way to work out, eat healthily, and live a balanced life to be physically fit. I wanted to take those same principles and apply them to conditioning the mind to be mentally fit. My goal is to help you achieve greater results. Because everything starts at the mind level, being mentally fit is a necessity to all. Who can't benefit from hands-on instruction?

All you need to do then is show up and be willing to work. The first half of the book details the warm-up, stretching, mind composition, mental weight loss, the building of mental strength, and the gaining of mental endurance. The second half of the book is comprised of steps to reach a full life. By employing the steps and advice in this book, you will be training your mind so that you can be a better, successful, and mentally fit person. As I've already begun this journey, I would like for you to join me as I become your personal trainer for your mind.

Part 1:

Exercise Stations

- The Warm-Up: Take a Lap with Me
- Stretching the Mind: Full Range of (E)motion
- Mind Composition: Pull Out the Measuring Tape and Mind-Fold Caliper
- Losing Weight: Step on My Mental Scale
- Mental Strength: Bench-Press Your Problems
- Mental Endurance: Breathe Inspiration to Sustain Life and Health

Station 1—
The Warm-Up: Take a Lap with Me

"Every great performance requires intense warm-up."

In grade school, we all took physical education. The instructor of the hour would blow his or her shiny, polished whistle and command, "All right, take a lap!" and we would say, "Aww man!" to ourselves, take a deep breath, and exhale forcefully. Most of us didn't like to take warm-up laps, but maybe you were the person who enjoyed every moment of gym class and couldn't get enough. Whichever person you may have been, the idea is that we all had an attitude toward warm-ups.

The warm-up readies the body for strenuous and physical activity by increasing the core temperature of the body, as well as increasing blood flow. These occurrences prepare the body for optimal performance. Without the warm-up, the body is hindered from performing well. This is also very true for the mind. If we don't warm-up before mental activity, such as creative thinking, we may just pull a neuron. This is completely a joke, but to have an appreciation for limbering up the mind, we have to understand the strenuous activity of creative thinking.

Some people feel differently about what creative thinking is. My idea of creative thinking is simply a series of definitions beginning with the word *create*. *Webster's New Explorer Dictionary* defines *create* the following way: "to bring into being, make, or produce."[1] Combined with this definition is the definition

> Creative thinking is described as forming mental pictures in the mind by way of reflecting and pondering, which produces, makes, and brings ideas into being.

for *thinking*, which is "to form or have in the mind, to reflect on or ponder, or to form mental pictures."[2] By combining these two definitions we come to the explanation of creative thinking. Creative thinking is described as forming mental pictures in the mind by way of reflecting and pondering, which produces, makes, and brings ideas into being.

One great example of creative thinking can be found in the inventor, Walt Disney. Walt Disney's idea for his famous theme park, Disneyland, was birthed by watching his daughters play at a small amusement park. While there he noticed how worn out and filthy the small amusement park was. He also saw that from a distance the park seemed very interactive, but as he approached closer he saw that it was the furthest from the truth. Thus, he began to ponder and reflect on what it would be like to have an interactive and clean amusement park. From using his mind to reflect and ponder on how to make a better amusement park, he produced and brought into being a new idea that many people still enjoy years later.

Like Walt Disney, my typical warm-up in support of preparing my intellect, is the act of reflection and pondering. At every level of competition, the warm-up is very important, whether it's physical activity or mental activity. Singers warm up their voices before a performance; those in the orchestra tune their instruments and go over

4

their musical scales, and actors and actresses warm up by rehearsing lines one last time. No matter the activity, if optimum performance is what you're looking for, a warm-up is what you need.

After graduating from college, where I was also an athlete, I began to take a closer look at the intricacies of and correlations between sports, physical activity, and life. Understanding that the mind can be trained and enhanced is vital to learning how to warm it up, which we must do if we want it to

> The warm-up is the process of familiarizing ourselves with a person, idea, thought, or thing.

perform well. The warm-up is the process of familiarizing ourselves with a person, idea, thought, or thing. You can probably think of a time when you needed your mind to work at its best, but somehow, it seemed like it wouldn't. Can you remember such a time?

I can give you one of my moments, which involves this book. One night, I sat down to start the writing process. It was twelve o'clock in the morning, and I felt I had ideas as I sat in front of my laptop, but somehow, they didn't find their way onto the screen. My mistake was that I tried to jump right into the writing and thinking process without a proper warm-up, and that is a no-no.

I struggled for the first few minutes, and since I'm somewhat of a perfectionist, I noticed myself constantly hitting the backspace bar. All of that time wasted when I could've warmed up to get my juices flowing! I tried to get my mind to do something that it wasn't ready to do, and that was to think creatively. I had been mentally unconstructive all day, and then I expected my mind to produce optimal results from little preparation—not to mention how late it already was.

Just like I did, most of us want to skip the warm-up and get right to producing results. So how could I have done this differently and warmed up before I started the creative thinking process? Just as Walt Disney pondered and reflected on how to make a better amusement park, I could have pondered on the ideas that I wanted to convey, and reflected on what those ideas meant to me and my message. Thus, doing so, my mind would warm-up to think creatively. By using my mind to ponder and reflect on current concepts and ideas, as Walt Disney had also done, I was able to gather an eclectic array of ideas, which usually lead to new ideas.

You may be saying, "Wow, dude! Haven't heard that one before. Where is the magic wand? I want to know how to make something appear from thin air." Sorry to tell you, folks, but there is no magic wand. There is no secret formula to getting your mind into a state of readiness to come up with great ideas. Through my studies, I've found this to be accurate. However, I will disclose to you this one secret. All of the great thinkers and innovators, believe it or not, have received inspiration from one another to embellish old ideas, and possibly form new ideas.

From reading other people's bright ideas and reflecting upon them further, great thinkers were able to come up with even greater ideas. All the greats do it; they've just been able to keep a tight lip about where they get their inspiration. In our society, we've become complacent, and some of us either refuse, don't know how, or feel that we don't have enough time to think creatively or constructively. We become bogged down with television and the Internet and forget that any one of us could be the person with the next great idea. Great ideas come about by great thinking, and great thinking only comes with a desire to capture the great thoughts of others.

> By thinking on great thoughts, we become a conduit for great thoughts.

The mind is a wonderful thing. The great discovery, which we've known about for thousands of years, states that whatever we think about the most, we become. This is clearly why the Bible says to think on these things: "Finally, brothers, whatever is true, whatever is noble, whatever is right, whatever is pure, whatever is lovely, whatever is admirable—if anything is excellent or praiseworthy—think about such things."[3] By thinking on great thoughts, we become a conduit for great thoughts. This is because we've warmed up, loosened up, and limbered up our minds for such thoughts.

Your intellect has to brood over (sitting or focusing on an idea keeps it warm and of primary importance, which allows it to mature until it's ready to hatch into a new idea) the intellect and thoughts of other great thinkers if you have a desire to birth great thoughts of your own. Meaning, you really have to take a concentrated effort to think on the great thoughts of others. So ask yourself this question: "To what do I give my attention the most?" This is important to discover, because we may be warming up to unconstructive thoughts without realizing it. These thoughts that are unconstructive will lead you to the development of your own unconstructive thoughts.

An example of this can be seen in the workplace. Have you worked with someone who does a minimal amount of work, but still gets paid the same amount as you at the end of the week? You're a hard worker and come to the realization that you're doing twice as much as they are, and receiving the same amount of money for it. So you begin to entertain this thought in your mind: *Why should I continue to work hard when, they don't, and we get paid the same amount each week?* By focusing your attention on this thought, you slowly transform into a slacker just like the person in question.

There is no escaping this law. Unconstructive thinking hinders most people and, because of this law, many people become what they don't want to become, and in this case that is unconstructive. This is why great thinking has become a lost art. Seldom do we constructively think on the thoughts of other great thinkers, which make reading of top importance in warming up the intellect. Someone may ask, "Why is reading so important?" Surely, reading helps us loosely understand the thought processes of an author. For example, if I would like to understand Dale Carnegie, the pioneer of self-help, I would read Dale Carnegie's books. But reading for mere entertainment is not enough. This is where we begin to really warm up. The following are questions to ponder while reading:

What's the focus of this book?

What am I looking to receive?

What have I received so far?

How can I make this information applicable to my life?

What similar thoughts do I have that can be enhanced by having read this material?

What causes this author to have this perspective?

I call it the art of studying great minds, which is better known as studying the psychology of great thinkers, and you don't need a doctor's degree to do it. Have you ever wondered why some people seem to be more successful than others? It's not because they were born that way—even though intelligence can lie in genetics, but even then someone can be very knowledgeable and have no wisdom. Successful people seek and crave wisdom, and they find it from people who have acted wisely in their lifetimes. So the term *warm-up* here can be used in the context of warming yourself up or familiarizing yourself with other individuals' thoughts, as in

So the term warm-up here can be used in the context of warming yourself up or familiarizing yourself with other individuals' thoughts.

the phrase, "Yeah, they're beginning to warm up to me," meaning building a relationship and becoming familiar with that person.

Warming Up to the Thoughts of Others

Here is an example to help you better understand this point. In the time period of an infant's development in which they begin to notice that they can possibly talk, they usually stare directly at the mouth of the person doing the talking. As they stare, you can see their little lips moving in the same way as those of the older person. They are shaping their lips to produce the same sounds as they are hearing. "Say, Da-Da." Adults try to accentuate every syllable, so that the baby can follow along. We can take a lesson from the little ones here, because this is how we warm up our minds to think great thoughts. We pay close attention to how the great thinkers thought. We stare right into their minds and try to figure out exactly what they were saying and thinking.

We shape our minds to theirs as we try to understand and comprehend, just as babies shape their mouths as they try to speak. We see that children learn to speak from an adult, but as the children grow, they develop their own way of speaking and conveying ideas. The adult was just the launching pad or the warm-up. The process is the same for us; by reading and thinking, or at least trying to think like successful people, we use their thoughts as a launching pad. Eventually, we develop our own awesome thoughts and ways of expressing ourselves.

During the process of writing this book, I developed the habit of reading a chapter or two of another book written by an author whose material I enjoyed. By reading the material of this author, I began to warm myself up to write my book (though still not nearly as good a writer as this author). Now, allow me to clarify. This was done in no way to steal or duplicate this author's ideas. The premise was to have this author's grammatical structure and word usage fresh in memory so that I could at least write a reader-friendly book. Knowing that this author writes reader-friendly and captivating books, I decided to use the style as a launching pad, although I still placed my own touch in my writings.

For two years while in college, I was president of the Fellowship of Christian Athletes, also known as FCA. I did fairly well, but I wasn't truly pleased with my performance as a speaker. One day, I asked our spiritual coach, who has a successful church, "Have you always been a good speaker?"

He shook his head and said emphatically, "Oh no, not at all." What he told me changed my perception of all great thinkers, speakers, and leaders. He said his whole life he had been an introvert, much like me, but what he learned was this one technique that I'll sum up in five words: what you read, you speak.

I began the process of reading as many books as I could to develop this trait and have become quite fond of it. Since you're reading this book, I'm sure you don't have a problem with reading, so encourage others to read as well. For the person who says, "Well, my job doesn't require me to do all of that reading. How can it help me in my life?" my response to that is that reading can help improve your awareness. It can also make

> Being informed will help you make wise decisions.

you a better all-around person. Being informed will help you make wise decisions.

There's always something that we can learn from reading that will not only improve our lives but those of others as well, as we may be able to inform them wisely by our newfound knowledge. Thomas Jefferson, the third president of the United States, is known to all as a great thinker, which would also mean that he was a great reader. If this is the case, there should be no wonder about how he authored one of the single greatest documents of all time: the Declaration of Independence. We have to realize that his thoughts didn't fall out of thin air. He read the writings of such people as John Locke, Isaac Newton, and Francis Bacon and constantly read the classic writings of Tacitus.

He modeled his life after the Roman philosopher, Marcus Tullius Cicero. Of course, he learned about the life of Cicero by reading. So the secret behind great ideas is to figuratively eat great ideas—of course in the mental concept of eating. Not to sound ghastly, but if you put enough books down the ole mind belly, something is bound to come back up. So, is reading about the lives and ideas of other successful people enough? It's a good start, but to really warm up for maximum benefit, your next step is to think by reflection and pondering.

We're Warmed Up

Ponder what you've read by thinking about how it relates to your life or world or about what you could draw from and connect to other ideas that you've read. Mingling two or more ideas, related or unrelated, may birth something new. Just as Walt Disney took his experience as an animator and combined that with his ideas on an ideal amusement park.

> Mingling two or more ideas, related or unrelated, may birth something new.

Presenting ourselves with quality questions assists in the enhancement of our reflecting. In John Maxwell's book, *Thinking for a Change*, he points out this one activity, which I associate with warming up the mind. He states, "The value you receive from reflecting will depend on the kinds of questions you ask yourself."[4] Many times, I've read something weeks earlier, and while reading something new, I have had an epiphany or new idea. The interesting thing about questioning and reflecting is that it's something we do every morning when brushing our teeth. (I hope we all do this every morning.)

Most bathrooms have a mirror above the sink where we have a clear view of our reflection. We cast our image in the mirror, and by doing so, we can see things that we otherwise may have missed. How embarrassing is it when we miss something because we forget to question or consult our reflection before going out? I hope you see the point here, and that is to understand that the importance of questions and reflection is to help us see things that otherwise may be difficult to see. Reflecting will also help us see things that we have missed. How does reflecting work?

180 Degrees of Order and Equality

Now that we're warm, allow me to show you how warming up can place you in the flow of acquiring new ideas or perspectives, by borrowing from my own experiences. One day, I was brushing up (warming up) on geometry—it's important to note that earlier in the week, I had been reading something about the pyramid structure of hierarchy. We know that a pyramid on paper is really a triangle because it is two-dimensional, but something struck me as I was studying geometry. I remembered that every triangle has a total of 180 degrees! You may be thinking, "So what's your point?" Well, the point in this case is that in any isosceles triangle, which is the makeup of any hierarchical diagram, each angle is approximate to 60 degree and three angles total 180 degrees.

This is the overall point, however: we also know that a straight line is 180 degrees. Although God created hierarchy for purposes of order, He never intended for one person to be viewed as a lesser human being than any other. We all have a role to play in this world, and if someone happens to be closer to the top of the hierarchy and someone else closer to the bottom, it doesn't mean that the higher one is better. We're all in the triangle of hierarchy, which is 180 degrees, and ultimately a straight line of equality. There should be a level of interconnectedness, love, and compassion between people in spite of hierarchy.

As a result, those who are fortunate to have a higher position have an obligation to be of service to those who are lower.

If you're having trouble understanding this concept, examine the diagram below. Some people may think that this isn't very creative at all, but it's one way of looking at things differently. And this is an example to show you how mingling two unrelated ideas can birth something new. There is a level of equality that exists because we are created by one God, and we all fit in the hierarchy in some way to do what we were sent to do (although we can forfeit this right). Therefore, no one should look down his or her nose at anyone else. No one is separate from the hierarchy.

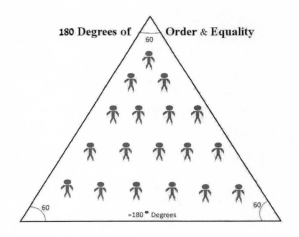

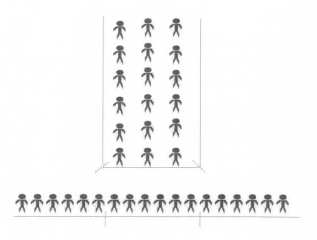

I hope this example helps you understand how important warming up the mind is. Only by warming up the mind can we use it to its optimal level. I would like to note however, that reading isn't the only way to receive information, although it's the chief way. We can listen to audio programs, attend seminars, be mentored by someone successful, or by becoming aware of our surroundings. The famous comedian Jerry Seinfeld, reportedly develops his material in this way. His brand of humor which ultimately is his creative way of reaching his audience is deemed, "observational humor." By being aware of what's going on around him, he is able to combine everyday occurrences with humor. Any of these methods is a good way to learn and a good way to receive information in order to develop your own ideas. Here is a simple plan to begin to warm up your mind.

As your personal trainer, I am now convinced that you understand the importance of reading and listening to successful people on a daily basis. As a result, I will get you started on your warm-up routine, so here is what I want from you.

Exercise Points

We are going to take a few laps.

1. First lap—Take a lap around your object of focus. How is this done? Read up on the literature specific to your focus. View online videos concerning your focus, or speak with someone who knows what you want to know. If you don't have a focus, you can read or listen to what interests you on a daily basis.

2. Second lap—Make sure that you are not reading or listening for mere entertainment but to receive something from the information. So be attentive.

3. Third lap— Question, ponder, and reflect. Try to find connections between what you have read or heard. It's more common in this process to connect and compare ideas than to contrast them.

4. Last lap—Whatever thoughts you have that strike you, write them down immediately or record them on a digital recorder. Don't rely on your good memory. Remember, great thoughts don't happen all the time.

Once you have warmed up sufficiently, we will go on to our next step in the progression, and that is the process of stretching. So when you're ready, I'll see you there. Okay, let's go! Take a lap! [Whistle blares.]

Station 2—
Stretching the Mind: Full Range of (E) Motion

"A muscle that is not properly stretched isn't only more prone to injury but is also an underutilized muscle."

After the warm-up, we should be ready for the stretch—the other thing most disliked about exercise. How many of us are guilty of skipping the stretching and moving right to the workout? We know it's good for us, but we dislike it with a passion. Why is it that some of us dislike stretching?

Well, mainly because it hurts, but also because it's monotonous. The commonly held belief in sports years ago was that stretching would hurt performance. Today, we understand that stretching will not hinder performance, but rather, it will enhance performance. Even for the average person looking to get into shape. However, this all sounds good and is well-known, but so many people still fail to include it in their workout.

Most people dislike the feeling of discomfort while being stretched.

They would rather avoid this pain. In the beginning the muscles are tense and there is only a limited range of motion that can be achieved. But if you've ever held a stretch long enough, you know that the muscles adapt and become more pliable.

The same is true for the mind. Most, individuals are initially resistant to stretching their minds. Stretching your mind will come in the form of welcoming the kind of change that accompanies discomfort. People are reluctant to welcome change because of the fear and the discomfort of the unknown. When change comes, they resist it, just like the muscles of the natural body resist the initial phase of a stretch. Just as the body, stretching the mind may be uncomfortable in the beginning, but if you continue to apply pressure, your mind will expand just a bit more.

The way we perceive and handle change is based on how that change makes us feel. Hence, if we can adjust the way we feel about the change in our lives we'll be better able to handle it. We'll be stretched to better assimilate to the change because we would have trained ourselves to stretch at a greater range of (e)motion. Simply meaning, we would be more emotionally mature. Emotional maturity is learning how to responsibly use our emotions for good. Using our emotions as a tool rather than allowing our emotions to use us. We'll talk more about emotion and its role in us occupying our purpose further in this chapter, but first let us go in and explore the reasons for why an individual loathes stretching. And see why one has to be stretched if an individual want success in their lives.

The Seen Give Voice to the Unseen

Determining what causes one to dislike physical stretching, helps in determining what causes one to dislike mental stretching. Physical stretching, which in action is immediately seen (by others) and immediately felt (by yourself), brings mental stretching, which is neither immediately seen (by others) nor immediately felt (by yourself), into broader understanding. The examples below describe how things that are seen with the naked eye assist in understanding the things that occur below the surface as the example above.

The body is a manifestation of the unseen things (to the naked eye) that comprise it, such as the strands we call DNA. In grade school we learned that DNA is a blueprint to the structure we know as our body. In essence, your DNA is a form of thought that describes you fully. Not how others perceive you but as you truly are objectively. DNA is an objective thought, and a thought can be an idea, plan, or opinion. In this case, DNA is just like a blueprint which is an architect's thoughts about how a building should look. God is your architect and His blueprint for you is your DNA. Your DNA decides how tall or how talented you will be. It decides whether your eye color will be green or dark brown.

It says whether you will be healthy or suffer from sickness. Your DNA, although not visible to the naked eye, makes itself known by how your body is objectively constructed. Here, with this example, it can be clearly seen that the body of an individual gives voice to the genetic code which occurs below the surface.

The next example comes from observing action and thought. Thoughts are unseen, but we are most definitely affected by them daily. Whatever thoughts we focus on will manifest in our actions. Our thoughts are spiritual in nature and our actions are physical in nature. Thoughts are spiritual because it was thought that created everything you see.

It was a thought from God who wanted to reveal His invisible attributes in what He physically created such as nature.[1] If you appreciate the idea of a blood bank, thank Dr. Charles R. Drew for his idea. If you're using a light to read this book, thank Thomas Edison for turning his thought into something physical, which is the light bulb. Each and every day, quite literally, we walk through the minds of other people without realizing it. Where do you think that pillow or that mattress you lay on at night came from? What about the clothes you wear.

Or the streets you drive on. Or even the door you open to go to work. None of it existed thousands of years ago. None of it existed hundreds of years ago. It all started as a thought. And as I said, thought has spiritual qualities, because like thought, spirit desires to manifest as God, who is spirit, manifested His nature through those things He made.

There is a spiritual law, which I like to call the law of expression. The law of expression states that it is the desire of spirit to be perceived by mind, expressed physically, and used purposefully. Spirit desires to be perceived through and by the minds of people. It desires to be expressed physically in the natural realm, and it wants to be used and

> The law of expression states that it is the desire of spirit to be perceived by mind, expressed physically, and used purposefully.

harnessed with and through specific intent. It has the desire to serve a purpose. This relates to us through the thoughts that we carry. How does this relate to our thoughts? Because thoughts, which are unseen, wish to be seen, expressed, and used.

These two examples assists in our understanding of how our bodies and the things that we do with our bodies will and can help us have a better understanding of how our minds work. The correlation between why we dislike stretching in the gym and why we dislike stretching in life can be appropriately reached. One can be readily seen, but the other seems to be more complex and hidden from view.

Comfort Zones

Stretching in the physical context elongates our muscles, and we become more flexible, but certain methods of stretching may also help with improving the power and explosion within our muscles

20

(plyometrics). This is important information to remember later. When speaking about life, it's difficult to aspire to any worthy goal if we do not stretch ourselves or allow ourselves to be stretched. As we've been speaking about, what is that one very important muscle that needs to be warmed up and now stretched? Yes, you have it: the mind. So here we are talking about the dreaded stretch or stepping out into dark territory, which is murky and scary at best.

Oftentimes, I have heard the phrase *comfort zone*. A comfort zone is exactly what it sounds like, a zone of comfort. We can get into a zone of comfort and not even realize it. I'm sure you've heard about the gymnasts or other athletes who usually perform their best when they are in the zone. This zone is a place in their minds where they are so intensely focused on the final result that that's all they desperately desire. For athletes, being in the zone is good but for others being in the zone, particularly the zone of comfort, may not be as good.

Most people know what it is to be in the zone of comfort. So intensely focused on desiring comfort that's all they want. Picture yourself entering into a crowded auditorium to hear the speaker of the night deliver their oration. You don't know if any friends are going to be there, but it's a possibility that they may. You pull the door open and step in. What is your first thought?

Better yet, what is your first action? If you're the average person you may walk slowly scanning the room looking for a familiar face. If after searching far and wide you can't find a familiar and friendly face your next step is probably to seek the most comfortable seat you can find. Not because the chair is comfy but because the people in the area you are most comfortable with.

What happens if we enter the auditorium and find absolutely no one we would feel comfortable sitting by? What are we to do then? Well, when we don't know anyone in the room, the next best person to sit by is ourselves. But that's not even possible. And I say this humorously.

Nevertheless, we see how desperate we are to feel comfortable. We are willing to sit by ourselves, as if that were possible. I'm not beating anyone down because, yes, I too suffered from this syndrome. If you're not the person who is the everyday extrovert and loves to make friends, you're more than likely going to search for comfort by being by yourself. Comfort is what holds many of us back and I believe that it's fair to say that we are not doing ourselves any favors if we limit ourselves in this manner. This manner being the way we disassociate ourselves from others in order to reach comfort.

Emerging from Our Comfort Zones

This is where stretching becomes important. We want to jump right to a thing, like making friends, but we fail to make ourselves friendly. We would rather be in the zone, and the only thing that we're focused on is ourselves and the desired result of being as comfortable as possible. To many, comfort is much too important. Comfort is not a bad thing, but when it interferes with our progress, it becomes the enemy.

For instance, think of the students in class who are afraid to raise their hands, because they don't know how their classmates are going to react—this is comfort as an enemy. Let me remind you, I played football in college. I raised my hand often, and oftentimes, when raising my hand to answer a question and participate, I was made fun of. I got teased by my teammates, but many semesters, I was on the dean's list. You may be well into your profession and may be in a meeting when there is a situation on which you aren't clear. Since no one else has asked any questions, you decide you won't either.

You decide that you'll just wing it. That's not a smart move. By seeking comfort an individual may tamper with their ability to be stretched. When one lets comfort prevent them from expressing their inner self, it interferes with personal development and progress. By asking, you may be the one who stands out in the boss's eyes, because you are showing that you care. We must learn to stretch in our lives and not be afraid of making a mistake or looking incompetent. What are other ways we can we stretch or be stretched?

It's always beneficial to have at least one good and close friend. This friend can become an awesome asset to your life. Some people hate the sound of rebuke or constructive criticism, but these words, given in a loving way, are what oftentimes will cause you to stretch and grow. Don't be afraid of the truth about yourself. I know it's frightening to know that we aren't as perfect as we'd like to think, but show me someone who is, whose name isn't Christ. We can fall into the comfort zone again by not wanting to know the truth about ourselves, because, as the adage goes, "The truth hurts."

Grow to be the person who looks for refinement. The person who doesn't mind being told that he or she is wrong is the person who doesn't mind progressing. I learned this lesson early. I found that it was better to listen to open rebuke and see if it applied to me rather than completely ignoring it altogether. If I want to serve my purpose I have to welcome discomfort. It's a comfortable place to hear exactly what you would like to hear about yourself, but growth usually doesn't accompany comfort. I'm not saying that it can't but it usually doesn't. Ask yourself with sincerity: is it possible for me to serve my purpose if I'm afraid to grow?

Whom can I help when I'm only focused on helping myself and sitting by myself? Growth and comfort are antonyms, but growth and discomfort are synonyms. What if Steve Jobs and Steve Wozniak had become comfortable with building their business in Jobs' garage and felt no need to grow? No one can say for sure, but I can guess that we probably wouldn't have all the witty innovations that came from that decision to grow. A personal experience from my life came when a friend of mine said that I needed to network more.

Networking? Even though I knew I needed to get out and meet new people, it was nerve-racking just thinking about it. So what did I do? I began to network and talk to people. Me, the introvert sparking up conversations with complete strangers! I was a grown man and still wanting to use the excuse, "My mom told me not to talk to strangers." That's only a joke, of course; however, in this time of my life, someone pointed out to me where I needed to grow, and I willingly accepted it as fact.

A great number of us aren't honest with ourselves. We know where we need improvement, but sometimes, it takes another person to come along and push us toward improvement, and then it's our duty to act. When stepping out of our comfort zones, it's excruciatingly painful, but with practice and persistence, we'll

> Progress isn't built on one big block. It's built on smaller separate but conjoining blocks.

find ourselves becoming more flexible and pliable to our surrounding environment. In the same fashion that we stretch our muscles in the gym, we should stretch our minds—slowly at first, with minimum range, and once that becomes easier, go a little further, and when that is easy, go even further until there is complete range of motion.

Progressing in this manner builds flexibility, and flexibility will eventually translate to power. Progress isn't built on one big block. It's built on smaller separate but conjoining blocks. Therefore, progress should be handled one step at a time. Over time, we'll have a grand edifice that we call success and growth.

Stepping Out of Tormenting Fear

Stepping outside of our comfort zone and onto the pavement of success starts with a decision, and that decision is in the following statement: "I will not let this fear bring me down or keep me from reaching my destiny." A while back, I was reading the Bible and began to think about the concept of fear. I had a question, and the question was, "If God didn't give us a spirit of fear, then why should we fear Him?" After prayer and careful analysis, God revealed the answer to me. The answer was that there are two forms of fear. There is tormenting fear, and there is reverent fear. Tormenting fear is designed to cause pain, doubt, anguish, and anxiety. Reverent fear is designed to cause peace, confidence, faith, and hope. The world operates under tormenting fear. This fear keeps us from reaching our destiny. Reverential fear is from God. It is the awe-inspiring deep respect He deserves. Each form of fear has a four-step process:

Tormenting Fear

Ignorance→Fear→Hate→Death

Reverent Fear

Knowledge→Fear→Love→Life

The first step is either ignorance or knowledge. In tormenting fear, the first step is always ignorance. When we lose sight of who we are in God and what God has created us to be, we lack the knowledge to become what we have the capacity to be. As the Bible states, in the book of Hosea, "My people are destroyed from lack of knowledge."[2] Or, in other words, they perish because of their ignorance.

The second step is tormenting fear. People are naturally afraid of what they don't know or understand. The third step is hate. If, for a period of time, a person continues to lack knowledge about a certain aspect of life, which often leads to fear, they then develop hate as a mechanism of protection. This

> People are naturally afraid of what they don't know or understand.

mechanism of protection begins defensively but can become offensive. When it becomes offensive it has the possibility of leading to the last step which is death. Let's pull up an example.

Bigotry is the result of the ignorance of a certain group of people or of a certain culture, and because this ignorance is prevalent, there is no empathy, therefore meaning fear isn't far behind. In other words, once fear sets in, hatred develops, and once hate develops, the next thing is violence, which often ends in death. To give another, lighter example, we can go back to the classroom. College students must be knowledgeable about their course work. If they aren't knowledgeable, they're ignorant of it, and if they have a teacher who loves pop quizzes, this is bad for them.

As a result of the students not knowing the information, they become fearful of going to class because of a possible pop quiz. After a while, if the students want to remain ignorant of the course work, they will also remain fearful of going to class, and then they'll begin to say things like, "I hate this class." More than likely, these students will come to hate the class so much that they'll stop going. Eventually, if this persists, the students will ultimately kill their grade and receive a big ole "F," which ironically rhymes with death. Now I know that this scenario might be a stretch, but you get my point.

Reverent fear is the exact opposite. If we know God and know who God made us to be, then we are knowledgeable, and this is a good first step. Next, would be the fact that we respect God, ourselves, and others, because we would then have an appreciation for life via our knowledge. As a result of our respect and appreciation for God and life, we then will love and not hate, and finally we will have life and not death, all because we made the decision in the beginning to be knowledgeable. I don't know about you, but I think I would like to have an abundant life full of good success. But we see that it all begins with a decision that must be made, and that is to be knowledgeable about who we are.

Expand Your Interests

I'm aware that we all have our own interests in life. We have our own hobbies and likes and things that we give our attention to the most. Allow me to share with you another way of stretching your mind. Take the time to submerge yourself into another area of interest that you may not have thought about looking into. If you enjoy science, you may take the time to research history, or if you are a musician, you may take the time to brush up on paintings or something far out there like motorcycles. This will cause you to grow in your life and become more knowledgeable about other things besides your current interests.

It'll be hard in the beginning to pull yourself away from the things that you enjoy doing, but we're working on stretching here, so it's okay to feel uncomfortable. If you can remember, earlier in this chapter, I said that stretching can improve both your flexibility and power. If you can, for a second, imagine a rubber band. Place one end of the rubber band around one thumb, and pinch the opposite end between the thumb and index finger. Draw it back as if shooting an arrow from a bow, and release it. Watch as it goes flying across the room.

What we have done here is demonstrate the ability to develop power from a stretch. The potential energy in the rubber band becomes kinetic energy once it's stretched to a certain point and released. The degree of the stretch determines the distance it will travel. Ah ha! Did you catch that?

That's the secret? How far we decide to stretch determines how far we'll go. As a result of stretching, power ensues. In my field of interest, which is sports and physical activity, I constantly hear

> How far we decide to stretch determines how far we'll go.

about the potential that athletes had resting inside of them. I know I've heard it spoken into my ear plenty of times. The potential that so many crazed parents, coaches, and sports analysts are referring to is the ability for those athletes to transcend their current level of play and go to the next level.

The potential that they have is the talent graced to them by God, but this talent occasionally isn't in motion the way it should be. You will hear the coach say, "I need more passion!" or "I need more focus!" or plainly enough, "I need more from you. I need you to live up to your potential!"

> This potential energy is manifested in how well these players do above what they have already achieved.

The coach will oftentimes do whatever it takes to motivate the potential in players to get it to move and have motion and become kinetic, manifested energy. This potential energy is manifested in how well these players do above what they have already achieved. Successful coaches have realized to get an athlete to improve their performance he or she has to move the athlete emotionally and not yell or curse unscrupulously. He or she has to stretch the athlete's ability to tap into their emotions. Here's another secret I'll share with you in a few blurbs. Potential energy in motion is kinetic energy, and kinetic energy is the perfection that you see coming from individuals who are skilled in their particular field.

Therefore, activated potential (talent) supercharged to a high degree (skill) is perfection. Also, it's important to note that emotion is energy in motion, which means that emotion is the catalyst to internal spiritual and mental movement. So to become that person who will translate potential energy into full-fledged kinetic energy or the closest thing to perfection, you must get that potential moving, and you do that by generating strong emotion in the form of passion.

Passion

Passion is the strongest emotion we have and for good reason. Passion can be used for purposes that will promote either good or evil, blessing or calamity. Passion is where we start to bring out the best in ourselves. Passion sets the potential in motion. Just check out all the greats in their respective fields; they all had one thing in common: passion! Nevertheless, we cannot evoke this strong emotion without first realizing the stretch. Where exactly does passion come from? And how does passion develop in a person?

Is it God given? Is it downloaded into our genetics? Or can we develop passion of our own? I've never known a person who had a passion for something and wasn't good at it. Now I'm not talking about the diehard sports fans. They're more like fanatics. I am referring to those individuals who have a great desire to enhance the lives of others by performing and refining their talents and gifts. So where does passion come from?

> The ones who have passion are imbued with strong feelings, enthusiasm, and love toward their object of affection.

Webster's New Explorer Dictionary defines passion as: "strong feeling ... LOVE; also: an object of affection or enthusiasm."[3] The ones who have passion are imbued with strong feelings, enthusiasm, and love toward their object of affection.

The Purpose Equation

The formation of passion is a mixture of a few ingredients, which include God-given ability, love for people, righteous anger or compassion, and the unknown factor. Or try this equation:

My passion or purpose = the unknown factor x ability + righteous anger or compassion x love

You can almost always find your purpose by using this equation, because usually, what you're passionate about is what you're purposed to do. Here, in this equation, "ability" is short for God-given ability, such as talents and gifts. God will supply us with the necessary tools in order to get the job done right. I believe it's important here on the other hand, to convey how important it is to take what you're talented at and turn it into a skill. Making your talents, skills, will gain you influence to the unknown individuals you're destined to reach. The late great pop singer, Michael Jackson, took his talent in dance and music and made it a skill. Many people can dance, but not many people could dance like Michael Jackson. He took his potential, added passion and love, and turned it into one of the closet things to ever come close to perfection, and look at his influence.

Righteous anger is anger that isn't unsatisfactory. We can determine this by what causes our anger or what fuels us to show compassion. If it's anger toward someone because of what that person has done to us, the majority of the time, it's unsatisfactory. We have to be careful to note that the anger that is directed to a person because of what he or she has done to someone close to us may also be unsatisfactory. Our loved ones are as close to us as we are to ourselves, so we have to be careful to judge rightly the cause of our anger.

I'll use Jesus as an example. He wasn't mad at the money changers in the temple because they were in His way; He was upset because the money changers were in the way of others reaching the path of truth, which would better their lives.[4] This is a perfect display of my next ingredient, which is love for people. You can ask anyone who is immensely successful if they like to help people; their answer will be a resounding, "Yes!"

God didn't intend for us to be successful in life without the help of other individuals. We show love to people by giving them the things they need. You find your purpose and passion when you find the

> You find your purpose and passion when you find the compassion and love to help people.

compassion and love to help people. Finally, the unknown factor is the thing that you feel righteous anger or compassion toward and the place where you know you want to supply something that is beneficial to effected individuals. The unknown factor is unknown because everyone will have something different.

More than likely, this will be accomplished through an extension of your abilities; this is how you will reach the unknown masses. I can use myself as an example. I love to write and speak. These are my strengths. I feel empowered when I can speak to people, give them advice, or allow them to read my writings. So, writing is my God-given ability.

I become righteously angry and compassionate when I see people who refuse to think for themselves but rely on other people to do the thinking for them. As you can see, my concern for people isn't selfish in any way, and since I am not directly benefiting, this anger is righteous. You may even be thinking, *Why do you care if people would rather do their own thinking or allow someone else to do it for them?* Well, that's just the love that I have for people. I want to share this by the extension of my gift of writing. Lastly, you already know what the unknown factor is, and that is helping people or that group of individuals to think like they have the ability and capacity to think. So you can see my passion and purpose blossoming as I identify these few things. To get to your passion and purpose, you cannot miss any one of these aforementioned ingredients.

Love should multiply the intensity of your righteous indignation or compassion, and once this happens, you can then add this to your ability to help your specific group.

So how does this translate to stretching and power? Using myself for an example, by using emotion, namely passion, I'm able to stretch to a greater range. By becoming emotionally mature (understanding what emotions were designed for), I've learned to be stretched to a greater range by harnessing my emotions which helps me reach people, hence the title, "Full Range of (E)motion." Now that I have been stretched to love people and have become more social, I now have the power in knowing what my purpose is. The best thing about this is that I'm not being hindered because of my old comfort zones. I decided to stretch, and now I have power. The same will happen for you, because through being stretched, you adopt power. There is no person who is more empowered than the person who truly knows his or her calling and purpose.

Failing to Stretch Results in Injury

So are you now willing to stretch? Are you willing to be stretched? Remember, success doesn't come to those who run from stretching. What generally happens to those individuals who fail to stretch before strenuous activity is they end up injuring themselves. We can make a direct comparison between life and strenuous activity. Life is strenuous, and if life hasn't become too taxing for you, then continue to live, and it will eventually.

I don't want to be the bearer of bad news, but I want to be truthful. If you don't take the responsibility of stretching your mind, you will eventually hurt yourself and pull up lame. In the area of athletes' play, they have the ability to recuperate after a strained or pulled muscle, but in the real world, second chances are not as common when the mind hasn't

> If you don't take the responsibility of stretching your mind, you will eventually hurt yourself and pull up lame.

been properly stretched. Tell yourself that you love to be stretched, and you will become flexible. Remember this bit of information: a flexible muscle is a more powerful muscle, so stretch forth your mind and develop the power to push yourself vertical.

Okay, now it's time to apply what we've just learned. It's time to stretch. Follow the stretching instructions below, and I'll meet you over in Station 3 to discuss your composition and what we'll need to work on.

Exercise Points

Each exercise should be performed daily.

Stretch your mind as much as possible each day.

1. First Stretch Exercise—Read something informative and uplifting each day.
2. Second Stretch Exercise—Smile and be friendly. Be of good cheer each day. Try not to walk by a person without giving a friendly greeting. Think of something each day for which to be happy and grateful.
3. Third Stretch Exercise—Sit in the front row or by someone you do not know, but use good judgment with this one. Don't sit by a grouch.
4. Fourth Stretch Exercise—Become acquainted with different interests that won't detract from your life but add to it.
5. Fifth Stretch Exercise—Identify your ability, passion, and purpose. This may take some time, and it'll definitely stretch your thinking.
6. Sixth Stretch Exercise—Take steps toward fulfilling your purpose.

Station 3—
Mind Composition: Pull Out the Measuring Tape and Mind-Fold Caliper

"To think positively only is not enough for the attainment of personal achievement if works have been forsaken."

Body composition is the ratio between fat mass and other fat-free tissue mass, such as muscle, bone, water, and organs. Essentially, it's your body makeup in totality. When we perform physical exercises, the intent is not only to improve our health but also to change our body composition. We want to actually look healthy, not just feel healthy. So we work to exhaustion by jogging, running, or climbing on the Stairmaster for a few hours. Whatever the method of changing our bodies, we want to see results. We want to see the weight on the scale and the inches around our waist decrease.

Like the body, the mind also has a composition ratio, however not comprised of fat mass and other fat-free tissue mass. The mind ratio I'm referring to here is your percentage of mental strengths compared to mental weaknesses. To segue into our topic, the question to muse over is: *What is my mind made up of? What is my ratio?* I hope it's constructed with more strengths than weaknesses. A person of success has more mental strengths than they do weaknesses. This is what makes a successful person's mind composition healthy.

In this station, we'll focus on the mental strengths, and later, in station 4, we'll converse about the different causes of mental obesity which are mental weaknesses. We'll also identify how to lose the weight that causes mental obesity.

Active Affirmations

Both positive and negative affirmations are key components of creating the mind's composition. An affirmation is an assertion that is a biased truth. You repeat this biased truth to yourself whether verbally (speech), non-verbally (body), or by thought (visualization), and by repeating this biased truth overtime you become what you are asserting yourself to be. The reason that I consider active affirmations to be biased truths is because an affirmation is anything that we affirm as being true. If you affirm yourself as being smart, or if you affirm yourself as being unintelligent, you're right. You are what you believe you are. Most motivational speakers and success coaches will preach the strength and power of affirmations until they're blue in the face. These experts know of their power and effectiveness.

The intent behind an affirmation is to transform your mind from what it is to what you want it to become, in regards to gaining positive strengths and losing negative weaknesses. Remember seeing those before and after pictures from a physical health ad promising you the same results? What you're seeing is the body composition of the person changing, no matter how true it is. Take the time now to take mental before and after snapshots of your mind. What weaknesses or mental characteristics would you like to lose?

What strengths or mental characteristics would you like to gain? In your mind, visualize these characteristics. Visualizing the after picture is a form of affirmation because by thought you're affirming to yourself this is who you are and how you see yourself. What you see as the after picture of yourself, meaning after losing your weaknesses and gaining strengths, is what you'll be affirming as truth. For instance we can use verbal, non-verbal, and thought for this illustration of an active affirmation.

Let's say we want to meet twenty people each month for the purpose of networking along with growing confident and becoming more professional. Be sure to be as clear as possible about what you want to accomplish because affirmations and clarity are fraternal twins. It's hard to birth one without the other, so when making an affirmation, be specific about the desired outcome or result. So, then our outcome is increasingly becoming more confident and professional while meeting twenty people each month. The next thing to be mindful of is that each statement should begin with "I am" or "I." Saying "I am" or "I" is telling our mind this is something that it has to do and it has no option but to obey. The affirmation should also be in the present tense with as short but as clear a thought as possible.

Our affirmations would sound something like this: "I am a professional, confident networker. I eagerly meet new contacts daily." Now, as you repeat this—or rep this—over time, your mind will begin to take the shape of that of a professional, confident networker who is eager to meet new contacts daily. This form of affirmation is verbal, but we can also assume the physical disposition of someone confident by walking with our head up and being the first to introduce ourselves. This is non-verbal but nevertheless a very effective affirmation technique. And of course the last technique is to visualize ourselves as the statement says. In this case it's being confident and professional. These techniques are guaranteed to work every time when used with diligence.

One key point, however, is when we work out in the gym, if we want the best results quickly, we must work with intensity. The same is true here; to gain fast results, we must be active, intense, and especially dedicated. What I mean by active and intense is that we want to refrain from reciting our affirmations with a lack of zeal or enthusiasm. Remember those personal trainers in the gym? What is their usual disposition? Aren't they enthusiastic and encouraging? You are your own personal trainer, and you are the one conditioning your own mind. So you must be enthusiastic.

Enthusiasm has a purpose that lies in how the subconscious mind operates with strong emotion. In short, the subconscious mind is the part of the mind that controls everything without our direct interaction, such as the natural processes of the body, our instincts, and habits. Emotion is what places our subconscious mind into a sponge-like state that prepares it to receive pertinent information. Just like when you're startled, instantly that emotion of fear sends a signal to your subconscious mind and your subconscious mind decides if you should fight or flight.

> Enthusiasm has a purpose that lies in how the subconscious mind operates with strong emotion.

Our subconscious mind is designed to protect us, so when we evoke an intense emotion, our subconscious mind comes running to the scene soaking up the information to see what is wrong and how it can serve. Depending on the emotion, any past stored events similar to our recent encounter will metaphorically send our subconscious mind storming through its file cabinet. It then rises and takes over the show.

For instance, let's say we're playing baseball and someone throws the ball to us. The ball misses our glove and smacks us in the eye. Intense pain shoots throughout our eye, and we're in agony. So because of this pain and strong emotion, our subconscious mind stores this information so the next time someone throws us the ball, we may be apprehensive in catching it. If we don't work through this apprehension, it'll become ingrained in our subconscious mind, and thus it will become a part of us and guide us.

As a result, when reciting our affirmations, we must be active so that our subconscious mind is up and paying attention, learning how to best serve us. Our subconscious mind's greatest desire is to serve and protect us. We might as well train it to serve us with positive results and protect us from mediocrity. In stating our affirmations, we want to focus on the positive and not the negative. We want to use proper technique in our delivery. We should feel emotionally invigorated and filled with joy as we recite our affirmations.

> Our subconscious mind's greatest desire is to serve and protect us. We might as well train it to serve us with positive results and protect us from mediocrity.

As I've alluded to earlier, affirmations are similar to lifting weights, or for a more specific example, it's like performing dumbbell curls. Dumbbell curls build the front part of the upper arm, the muscle of the arm that is flexed when we say, "Make a muscle." As we rep this particular exercise, it stimulates the muscle, and as time passes, it begins to change form and take shape. It will begin to look stronger, more toned, and firmer.

By repetition and stimulation, we have caused it to take on a different shape. Affirmations, in much the same way, are repetitive exercises in the form of positive statements. After time has passed, your mind will begin to take on a different shape. It'll become stronger and firmer. This is a positive side effect of affirmations, but there can also be negative side effects.

Negative affirmations repeated over time will cause the mind to take the shape that is consistent with failure. Either way, we are strengthening our minds to be either a success or a failure. We are conditioning them to be successful or we are conditioning them for failure; the choice is up to us.

Negative Affirmations

"I am never going to be successful."

"I fear what my future holds."

"I am a loser."

"I should worry because nothing is ever going to change."

Positive Affirmations

"I am overjoyed because of my success."

"I am courageous and more than a conqueror."

"I operate in power, love, and have a sound mind."

"I am thankful for what God has blessed me with."

"I have a heart to give."

"I am passionate and enthused about my destiny."

"I focus on what is good and of virtue."

"I have favor with people and God."

"I am wealthy because I remember the Lord who has all power."

"I feel like today is a day to rejoice in."

"I have wisdom and understanding, which is like a wellspring."

As we can see, I decided to write more positive affirmations than negative affirmations. I also placed the negative affirmations first and the positive affirmations last. I did this because our minds tend to gravitate toward negative statements more easily than toward positive statements. Reciting affirmations is a matter of repeating enough positive statements to cancel and replace the entire negative repertoire. I must point out that the book of Psalms in the Bible is a book filled with positive affirmations. In this book, King David is seen reciting statements continually about the protection of God, the justic and the strength of God, along with other things.

This is one obvious reason to explain the success of King David when considering the circumstances and trials he faced. Although he went through much and saw much, he always kept a positive attitude by repeating positive affirmations. By continuing to believe in what he was reciting, he prevailed in the end.

Thinking with Clarity and Intensity

When we think about clarity, we may think of the term *crystal clear*. Some of us probably have tried the following experiment in class while in grade school. We shine white light through a prism. What happens? The white light is broken up into different colors (ROY G. BIV).

When we think intensively with crystal clearness, it's like passing our thoughts through a prism. This is significant because it causes us to view things in a different light and in different colors. We are given a

> When we think intensively with crystal clearness, it's like passing our thoughts through a prism.

brighter view of what wasn't as clear in the beginning and also that which wasn't easily seen or distinguishable. This is how clear our affirmations should be; they should be clear enough that greater vision will result, leading to ideas that will help us reach our goals.

Goal Setting

Goal setting is another important aspect of the mind's total composition. Whether we realize it or not, goal setting is a part of our daily lives. No matter if we set intentional goals or if we set unintentional goals, we all have set goals. It's important to set intentional goals, because if we don't, our minds will, by default, set goals for us, and these default goals are usually negative. The mind was designed to work, and its greatest desire is to serve.

Generally, if we do not give our mind constructive work, it will become destructive as a result. All things in existence have a purpose to serve, and our mind serves the purpose of serving us, but if we decide not to use it as it should be used, it will, on its own, begin to engage in destructive activity. For example, if we take a look at a large number of children in the inner-city environment, we can see that their minds are not stretched and aren't given over to constructive thought and behavior solely because of their environment. As a result, their minds will, by default, set goals for them. Usually, these goals are destructive in nature.

To understand how amazingly powerful our minds are, think about this analogy. In any James Bond (also known as 007) movie, James had a gadget wizard named Q. Q's specialty when designing a stealth weapon for James was to also install a built-in destruction mechanism. He did this so in the event of his technology falling into enemy hands, it would self-destruct, to prevent the enemy from benefiting from its technology. Well, if we look at how the mind is designed, we can see it is a fine piece of hardware.

It was designed for only purposes that would result in good and positive outcomes. When it falls into enemy hands, such as fear, doubt, anger, or hate, it turns on its self-destruct mechanism. Is there any other reason why thinking of fear, being doubtful, or having feelings of anger or sheer hatred usually leads to the destruction of the person's dreams or the life of the person? The person's mind will find a reason to mess things up. This, of course, is unintentional.

This is the point I'm making about the mind setting unintentional goals. This process of self-destruction isn't readily seen, but the process is set in place and the clock is ticking. Just think of the evil that has been perpetrated behind the mind of a genius. No evil genius lasts for long, though, because of the self-destruct mechanism. Although their goals are intentional, their goals seldom lead to positive outcomes, which sets the self-destruct switch. Some commit suicide. Others become prideful and take a wrong turn, and still others go insane. Therefore, we need to set not only intentional goals, but also goals that will lead to a positive and good outcome.

Heart

Many have heard this saying, "Your attitude determines your altitude." If you haven't heard this saying, allow me to tell you what it means. The way we think about others, our environment, ourselves, and God forms our attitude, and our attitude determines how high we will go in life. Our attitude is what holds together our affirmations

> The way we think about others, our environment, ourselves, and God forms our attitude, and our attitude determines how high we will go in life.

and our goals. If affirmations and goals were paper, our attitude would be glue.

To take this a step further, our attitude in some ways is synonymous with our heart, even though our attitudes don't cover the full spectrum of what a heart is. The heart is the component of our inner being in which we truly believe how we feel about others, how we feel about ourselves, how we feel about our environment, and how we feel about God. When we add these four categories with strong emotion, we come up with the condition of our heart. When someone makes reference to the heart in the context of emotion, we instinctively think about the heart in our chest. We know that this isn't the heart that we feel with, but instinctively, this is what we envision.

The heart that we feel with is not located in the chest but in the brain, which essentially is a component of the mind. The heart is located here, because this is where we think and decide how we will feel about others, our environment, ourselves, and God. One important thing to realize about the heart is that when we were conceived in our mother's womb, God didn't give us a heart; He only gave us the capacity to construct a heart. Why do I say this? Well, a child isn't born with a biased slant on life.

Children develop their views of life by the thoughts that they are subjected to and the thoughts that they entertain. Our attitudes are formed by our environment. They are not predisposed to us through genetics. So then it is safe to say a heart is constructed. When speaking of forming something, we can allude to the thought of building a structure. If God has given us the ability to construct our own hearts, then it would be wise of Him to give us tools with which to build, and He has done just that. God may not have given us a manufactured heart while we were being fashioned in our mothers' wombs, but He did give us manufactured tools with which we can labor and build.

These tools can be found in our toolshed, which is called the *soul*. Our soul houses our tools—the mind (intellect), the will, and the emotions. These three tools are what we use to construct our own hearts. Our chief tool is our mind, because it is the mind that controls everything else. The will is the servant to the mind, and the emotion(s) is the engine that moves the will and mind into action.

Emotions push the mind into the direction that it thinks it can go and take our will where it is willing to go. Our heart is a result of the mind, the will, and the emotions working together to construct and build. But that's not the end. In order to build, we'll also need building material. Ask any contractor and they will tell you that in order to build, you need tools, material, and labor.

So you're asking, "What is the material that we use to build our

> Emotions push the mind into the direction that it thinks it can go and take our will where it is willing to go.

hearts?" The material used is found in our environment. Our environment consists of the four things mentioned earlier, and that is other people, ourselves, God, and our general surroundings. There are many different things we can construct a heart for, and we can also construct a heart based on negativity or positivity, which are negative attitudes, positive attitudes, or negative beliefs, or positive beliefs. And, although a heart is often constructed by more subtle means usually without our knowing and consent (the belief-system we were raised under or major events usually negative that happened in our lives), we'll use direct language here to construct a heart. For instance, our heart is formed when we look into our environment, activate our mind tool, and say enthusiastically and believingly:

"Hey, I *believe* I can change and make a difference."

"I *think* I can get out of here and be something."

"I *know* I can be something better."

Or we can say antithetically:

"I don't *think* I can do any better than this" (and this is sometimes the problem because we don't think).

Then we use our will tool and say, I either *will* to change or I *will* to stay the same.

"I *will* change."

"I *will* change because I know I can change."

"I *must* change."

Or we can say antithetically:

"I *will* to stay the same; I will not change" (usually reinforced with an excuse).

After we think we can change and will to change, our next move is to find an emotion to bring about change. Our emotions push us to where our mind wants to take us, whether it's to be better or to stay the same, and our emotions enforce what we have as our will.

After we complete the task of thinking and willing, we then *feel* like we can be better, and we say:

"I have the *passion* to make a difference and to improve."

"I *feel successful*, and I am *happy* and *thankful*."

"I have the *drive*, and I am *hungry* for improvement."

Or we can say:

"Well, my momma didn't do anything. My daddy didn't do anything. My family didn't do anything. I'm not that smart, so why should I think I'll do anything?"

The emotion that is evoked here is self-pity, which leads to self-centeredness, feeling sorry about your situation, low self-esteem, and self-degradation. As I said, our emotions will push us where our mind wants to take us, even if it's negative. Usually, what we already have in our mind will call in an order for what form of emotion we need to get the job done.

It's important to note however, the greatest emotion that we have is passion. Passion is what moves us into our destiny.

I would like to point out that during most seminars that are designed to motivate, what usually happens is a great amount of emotion is generated, and we leave heading toward our destinies full steam ahead. The only problem is that our motion must be sustained by our emotions. Remember Isaac Newton's law of motion: a body will stay at rest until acted upon by another force. Our mind will only think it can do something until we actually will ourselves and add positive motion or emotion behind our thought, and we must keep this (e)motion constant. Earlier, I gave a brief description of how the tools perform to construct a heart. Again:

The heart is simply formed by the soul or our tools manipulating our perception to form what we truly believe about ourselves, others, God, and our environment.

I'll repeat it again in a different way; the heart is the place where our deeply seated beliefs, strong feelings, and true convictions are stored. It is the place where we are truly convinced. If all of our lives we were told that the sky is red, no one could convince us that it is blue because this is what we truly believe in our hearts. If we believe with our hearts, this is evidence of truly believing something. We can believe something with our logical mind but may not be truly convinced by it.

I may believe one football team is better than another, but by next year, I may change my mind. However, if I have a favorite football team, no one can convince me to go against my team, because I have *built* a heart for my team. I truly think that my team is the best no matter what their record says.

So let us reason:

If the heart is a place of thinking and housing our convictions, and if convictions aren't easily broken, then the heart can be likened to a mind-set or a mind that is set in its ways, because thinking originates in the mind. The reason I say this is because when we construct a heart for something, our opinion of it isn't easily changed. For the sake of combining these points, I believe it's important to recap here what a heart is. The heart is the component of our inner being in which we *truly* believe how we feel about others, how we feel about ourselves, how we feel about our environment, and how we feel about God. What we believe is true frames our heart. Since the heart is really a part of the mind we can also conclude that a broken heart is simply a broken mind-set. Just think about it in the context of a relationship with another person.

We use our *soul* or our tools to build a relationship with someone.

Wouldn't you say we use our soul to build a relationship? We build a heart for that person by concluding what we think about him or her is true. We *will* ourselves to believe that what this person has told us is true, and we also will ourselves to love this person. This is where a relationship begins to become a sacrifice.

This is why I believe love is a choice and not something that falls out of the sky at random. Lastly, our emotions come into play, and we begin to feel happy to be around that person. We begin to feel energized, and if that certain person is special, we may get "butterflies." These emotions reinforce what we think about this person as well as help us reinforce our will to love him or her. Essentially, what we have done here is construct a heart for this person, and this heart is in our possession, but we share it with that person in particular. Now, this isn't to say that emotion is what love is based upon.

Love is built on a decision that is enforced by an emotion to fulfill that decision. As stated, we share the heart that we build specifically for that person with that person. Have you ever heard people say, "I gave you my heart?" Well, this is what they were referring to, the building and sharing of their heart. They're sharing their deepest feelings and beliefs with this person who is now anchored in their convictions. So, this is why it's an important fact to consider that a heart is easily broken.

A heart is held together by what we believe to be true. When what we believe to be true turns up to be false, our hearts say, "Well, my only duty was to house and guard your truth, but now since the truth is not really the truth, what do I have to guard?" After this discourse, the heart we have built for this specific purpose of guarding and storing this specific truth is no longer needed, and it expires itself. It cracks and crumbles; it breaks.

Before I go on, I would like to share a story about my childhood years. My father has worked construction for as long as I can remember. He is also a phenomenal carpenter. I can remember when I was in elementary school, maybe around kindergarten or first grade. My parents decided to pour a slab of concrete in the backyard. I remember coming home excited because I wanted to see the big cement truck, but by the time I got there, my dad had already finished pouring the concrete and smoothing it out.

It was already in the process of curing or drying, but my mom did something that can still be seen to this day. She took a stick and on the edge of the slab, she carved my two older sisters' names and my name. It's still there years later. The reason I gave this illustration is because I wanted to give a picture of how our minds work. When we first go somewhere new or meet someone new, the beginning stages of the new relationship are like the pouring of the concrete.

As we become more acquainted with our environment and new people, we begin to smooth out different facts about them and their personalities and characters. In our environment, we learn new things about it, and we begin to formulate an opinion. After a while, the things that we have learned begin to cure, and the learning of these new facts is similar to carving or etching names into drying concrete. Down the line, we'll develop a solid foundation of what we think we know about our environment or the person. However, what if my mom had spelled one of our names wrong?

There would be nothing that she could do, unless she broke up the concrete and laid down a new slab. As I said earlier, this is what happens with our hearts. If we find something that is residing in our hearts to be incorrect, the best thing to do is to break it up and start over. Ironically, laying down concrete is easy; breaking up the concrete and removing it from its location is the hard part. Can you find the correlation?

Falling for someone is easy; breaking up with that person is hard, and removing him or her from memory is extremely hard. Just like removing broken concrete causes our bodies to perspire, so does breaking up with someone cause our souls to perspire in the form of tears. Remember, the eyes are the windows to the soul—this is true. Tears are a way of purging our souls. Calming our minds, taming our will, and discharging our emotions-pulling the power cord to our soul. So now we know how a heart is built and we know how a heart is broken, now let's investigate how a heart is fixed or mended.

The way a heart is fixed all depends on our attitude toward the work. The work is the removing of the shattered pieces. We can either work to pick up the shattered pieces diligently in forgiveness and move on, or we can remove the old pieces and start afresh. However, we don't want to feel like the victim.

I once had a summer job on a construction site. There were times while working when I could've said, "What is my boss thinking making us remove this heavy concrete in this heat?" We can say, "What were they thinking doing this to me?" The best way to get through the work is to have a positive attitude no matter the justification or the pain. At this junction, you may be wondering why this discussion about the relationship between our hearts and others is relevant to mind composition. Well, I wanted us to have a chance to see that even those things we house in our hearts are also a part of our mental composition.

Our hearts make up a great deal of our mental composition. The majority of our mental obesity or mental fitness resides in the heart as the heart is the place that shapes our perspective. We don't view the world objectively, we view it subjectively, and the subjection of the world is filtered through our convictions. The heart is where we pull from to encourage ourselves in our positive strengths or negative weaknesses. And yes, it is possible to encourage yourself to be negative.

So if we're obese because of negativity then we're weak, but if we're fit because we focus on what's positive then we're strong.

Although it's extremely difficult to construct a strong heart when it's based on the vacillating details of this world, we can always depend on the constant truth of love. Love doesn't faultier. Thus, construct a strong heart based on love. By doing so, our mental composition will change drastically for the better. We won't just feel mentally healthy, but we'll also look mentally healthy in the form of spreading love and having passion to conquer our goals. It's extremely important to have the ratio of the heart's strengths at a greater percentage than weaknesses if we want to be mentally healthy for success. At this point, we should know that strength in the form of active affirmations, goals, and a positive heart, is what causes a successful life.

Exercise Points

It's time to bring out the measuring tape and the mind-fold caliper.

This is your examination:

1. Identify both positive and negative affirmations that you repeat every day, whether aloud, by body language, or by thought.
2. Identify your overall views on your environment, yourself, others, and God. This information will give indication to your belief system and disclose errors in it.
3. Begin to develop the habit of constructing daily goals, short-term goals, and long-term goals, and stick to the script as closely as possible.
4. Recognize your view of forgiveness in others. Do you hold on to every event you deem unfair? Do you excuse yourself for holding on to those things you classify as severe, or are

you the person who can forgive in all situations no matter the unfair deed done?

5. Begin to make your subconscious work for you and not against you.

6. Don't just think positively; think correctly. Are you thinking in this way? Do you align your will with what you think? Do you evoke emotion to accomplish the desired result?

Station 4—
Losing Weight: Step on My Mental Scale

"Fear, much like a tick, is always looking for a connection, so that it can suck away the life of your dreams. Ticks can carry parasitic agents, and so can fear."

Without fail, news publications and health magazines illustrate the concerns about the obesity rate in America. Fast-food restaurants and high caloric food intake with lack of exercise are the main causes of this epidemic. Although this is fact, would you believe me if I told you our overweight bodies are because of our overweight minds? Remember, everything starts at mind level. People are healthy because they choose to be healthy, and people are overweight because they choose to be overweight. We may offer excuses as to why a person is overweight, but we cannot excuse ourselves from the fact that we are stewards of our own bodies. So in order to deal with the obesity of the body, we first have to deal with the obesity of the mind.

Mental Calories and Carbs

We eat food for energy so that we can expend energy. One

important source of energy comes from carbohydrates or *Carbs* for short. Carbohydrates provide the body with a source of energy in the form of sugars. Just as we have clean carbs and junk carbs in food, we also have clean carbs and junk carbs in our mind food. And just as we consume calories for energy, we also consume positive or negative energy through good or bad mind food.

Every day, we're fed vast amounts of rubbish in the form of mental garbage calories from sources of bad mind food. From commercials to billboards to music, we are fed calories upon calories. Just think if we were able to count the number of calories our minds take in on a daily basis. I believe that the five-hundred calorie sandwich wouldn't be as appalling. When we think of it, calories are just another form of energy stored in the food that we are consuming. What are some of the things that society offers that are mentally unhealthy for us?

The Prospect of Fear

Our society offers the prospect of fear everywhere we turn. From the fear of terrorists to the fear of losing a job, fear is real and it's active. Different voices are speaking in the same manner, offering fear to those who will accept. We all, at some point in our lives, will encounter fear, but it doesn't mean that we have to struggle with this emotion. In order to be healthy, we have to take a look at the nutritional value of fear.

Fear isn't good for our health, but we willingly consume it daily, and this has proved to be deadly. Fear is the leading cause of death of dreams, according to the surgeon general of dream health. There isn't really a surgeon general of dream health, but there should be, because dreams are dying daily. Once fear spreads, it is very hard to subdue, but it is possible eventually to grab fear by the horns and bring it to subjection. Earlier, in chapter 2, we spoke about two forms of fear, and this form of fear falls along the lines of tormenting fear..

Being afraid to go after what you desire is a form of tormenting fear.

Just take a second and think of how fear has affected your life. Fear is a bully; it likes to push people around. It holds your dreams dangling over your head out of your reach. The good thing about bullies is that we know how to deal with them.

When we were children playing on the playground, bullies may have seemed big and intimidating to us, but as we got older, we noticed that most bullies suffer from insecurity. There are plenty of stories in which the victim and the bully themselves became good friends after the victim

> Bullies may look big and mean, but on the inside, they think they're small and incompetent.

learned how to deal with the bully. Bullies may look big and mean, but on the inside, they think they're small and incompetent, which is why they pick on children smaller than themselves. Adults bully other adults for the same reasons. Here are a few pointers to help you overcome the "fear bully":

- Action cures fear.
- If you stand your ground and isolate the bullies, they'll shrink in size.
- Change your perception of the bullies' strength.
- Confidence is a repellant to bullies. If you're confident, you'll never show up on their radar.

Take note of what you can do to take action to overcome your fear. What driving emotion can you evoke to persuade forward motion? If you're afraid of networking, the only way to overcome that fear is to speak to the first person. Once you get the inclination to go for it, don't wait too long, because hesitation over extended periods of time nurtures fear. Lose the weight.

Standing your ground and isolating the bully is a proven method to stop bullying. Of course, you may get thrashed by doing so, but if you stand up to the bully, it generally is the last time they'll harass you. Bullies get satisfaction in making people afraid of them, and fear gets satisfaction in making people afraid of it, but standing up to them both takes the fun out of it, and it'll bother you less. Fear tries to isolate you, so isolate it; find out what you're afraid of, why you're afraid of it, and work courageously to overcome that fear.

Sizing Up Fear

Fear has its place, like when we are standing on a cliff of a mountain. This fear is survival fear. It also runs along the lines of being knowledgeable, but the fear that holds us back from our dreams works in the opposite way from that of survival fear, in that this form kills instead of preserves. We have to learn how to size up our bullies, see them for what they really are. The bully who is picking on a child can only do so if that child allows it; in the same respect, fear can only have power if we invest power over to it.

Let's practice putting our fears into perspective. The truth of the matter is our power surmounts the power of fear. We have the ability to give power, and nothing can take our power from us unless we give it away. So we must understand our worth and our power and comprehend our strength over our bullies.

Do You Trust Yourself?

Trust is paramount in any relationship. Doubt is the worst thing to have in a relationship. Do you trust yourself, or do you doubt yourself? What do I mean? Well, some people don't think that they can stand up to a bully. They don't trust themselves, and this is the very thing that bullies, such as fear, prey upon.

Fear isn't the big bad wolf or

> Those individuals who are confident and trust in their strength and abilities will never show up on a bully's radar.

the crazed animal we like to think it is. Fear is an opportunist. It seeks people who are unsure of themselves, and it harasses them. Those individuals who are confident and trust in their strength and abilities will never show up on a bully's radar. Fear is a magnet to distrust and doubt. Therefore, we should develop the habit of going forth each day with confidence in the person God has made us to be, in the abilities God has given us, and in the strength that He has bestowed upon us.

Doubt

If fear is equivalent to consuming food that is poor in nutritional value, then doubt is the disease that follows. It's not possible to have doubt without fear. If you can rid yourself of fear, you can rid yourself of doubt. When we doubt, we are thinking that something is unlikely or we distrust somebody or something. You've probably heard the saying, "Don't be a doubting Thomas." This saying comes from the Bible. When the disciples tried to convince another disciple, namely Thomas, that they had seen Jesus after His death well and alive, Thomas doubted.

Thomas didn't doubt because he didn't believe; the problem was that he desperately wanted to believe, but the fear that Jesus may not have returned from the dead frightened him into doubt. In any case, fear comes before doubt. Doubt is dead weight and is detrimental to the health of your dreams. Our dreams are not able to grow in the presence of doubt. If you want to be agile and speedy in reaching your dreams, then you do not want doubt on your back. Lose the weight.

We must be confident in order to dispose of fear, but we have to be careful how far we take our confidence. Having confidence in ourselves is in vain if the confidence that we have is beyond our God-given ability to support. If we're trying to tackle something that is beyond our ability to control, then we are vain in our confidence. God has given us all a certain level of ability to get certain tasks done, and how well we do those tasks depends greatly on how well we can prepare and enhance the ability that we were given. Again, I say this to point out that the aim of being confident in yourself stops at the ability to function by your abilities alone.

We are to trust in God with all of what we believe and not to depend on our own knowledge, so there is a spiderweb of interconnectedness between having confidence in God and in our abilities. Believing that God will help us improve in our abilities is one way of depending on Him, but it starts with being humble enough to know we can't do it all on our own.

Discouragement

Webster's New Explorer Dictionary defines *discouragement* as "1: to deprive of courage or confidence: Dishearten; 2: to hinder from disfavoring."[1] I find it interesting that discouragement, fear, doubt, et cetera, are all related and are blood cousins feuding with the perfect love family consisting of confidence, trust, hope, et cetera. We know that it takes courage to pursue our dreams, but we're always fighting with discouragement on our way to successfully reaching our goals. This reminds me of the cowardly lion of *The Wizard of Oz* who was always discouraged. His battle was finding a way to gain courage. And as he found out, in order to walk in courage, we need to learn how to encourage ourselves.

Encouragement can come from an outside source, but the dominant flow of encouragement we experience is going to come from within ourselves, hence the play on words: (in) encouragement. Some days, the voices of our best friends, parents, or those influential to us may not be there, and we will be the only people who can deliver encouragement to ourselves. So we should learn how to encourage ourselves, and the way that we encourage ourselves is to look within and find those things that will push and drive us forward. Inside of all of us, there is an encourager who will remind us why we should keep going and striving.

The only trick is learning how to fine-tune that voice so that it can be heard over the voice of discouragement; this is done by giving the voice of encouragement the stage more often to practice its voice. Singers enhance their voices through practice and getting on the stage; they have to get on the stage and behind a microphone. The same is true here; give the voice of encouragement room and time to practice and improve its voice. Rent out studio time to it. Musicians use studios to record songs; your personal private studio is your mind.

We are prone to rent studio time to every negative and atrocious voice, so why not a voice that'll sell records and be a hit? On any record label, if artists aren't producing good music, they're considered dead weight and are released from the label. In the same manner, some voices in our mind's studio aren't producing good music, so we have to let them go; they're dead weight. Discouragement is dead weight. Lose the weight.

Excuses

Covering this topic is a must. Many of us deal with excuses at some point in our lives. We would like to think that excuses are our best friends, but excuses are only our friends if we decide to regress instead of progress. If we have progress in our lives, excuses will be absent. Some of us believe that excuses will protect us from ridicule, but secretly, excuses are ridiculing us. Behind our backs, they poke fun and mock us as they hold our success at bay. This is one set of bad apples that will make us morbidly overweight.

> We would like to think that excuses are our best friends, but excuses are only our friends if we decide to regress instead of progress.

We pile it on and feed ourselves with excuse after excuse, thinking that somehow, we will feel better afterward. However, we don't realize that every time we feast upon an excuse, we are exposing ourselves to this disease spreading. We have never seen a person who is successful take on excuses as a friend. We're the company that we keep. All failures have allowed this impersonator into their circle of trust, and this impersonator does its job.

It does what it was created to do, and that is to hold people back from their destiny. In its hand, it has a ball and chain with a lock and key. Whenever we get into a clutch situation, it is there to bail us out. We think, *Wow! Thanks for bailing me out of that one!* But we don't realize that same excuse that bailed us out will in turn confine us to its own prison. Why? Because we have become indebted for using its services.

When we allow excuses to drop from our lips, they fall to the ground as a treadmill waiting for our next step. As we walk, we find ourselves going nowhere. When we look around, we wonder, *After all of this walking, why is it that I'm in the same position?* Successful people see excuses as a weakness to which they refuse to succumb. Failures see excuses as cover from the sun. Those who generate excuses are afraid that they will fail, but the same thing that they want to avoid, they become.

So how do we excommunicate excuses? Well, first, we have to be willing to step up and take responsibility. If something isn't done right, then taking the criticism and making sure it is done right the next time is what a responsible person void of excuses will do. Most excuses are given because of our lack of attention to detail and effort. They are offered when we have not done something with excellence, but only halfway, or when we didn't plan ahead and think about the outcome.

For example, if I have a meeting across town and I need to be there on time, I should take certain things into consideration. What time should I leave? What kind of traffic may I incur? Do I have gas, or will I need to stop by the gas station first? When we take responsibility for our actions, we'll have no reason to befriend excuses for a bailout. Excuses are issued for the sole reason of not being responsible. So, let's exercise responsibility and lose the weight.

Selfishness

Selfishness is something we're taught to nip in the bud when we're children, but this teaching evades some of us. Haven't we seen children playing and noticed how nasty stinginess looks? The child is running around the playroom yelling that everything is his or hers. Yes, it's cute when they're small, but when they are in elementary school, it isn't as cute. It looks even worse on adults when it comes in the form of thinking everything is about them.

We like to call those individuals narcissistic. So let's take a look at this and see why being selfless matters in losing weight in order to be successful. Just take a look at some of the major success examples in the world. What you will see is that they are mentally in shape for success, because they don't carry the weight of selfishness. Most of them, if not all, like to share their wealth, whether it is knowledge, contacts, or possessions.

They may have a foundation or give support to an organization, but whatever it is, they're selfless. Honestly, out of all secrets, this is a major secret that seems as if it's shared with those who reach the level of immense success. When you are in the multimillionaire and billionaire club, the technical name for giving is *philanthropy*. Even though I said that this is a secret, I was being facetious, because giving is plastered throughout many inspiring books. Whatever you would like to call it—sowing and reaping, karma, what goes around comes around, cause and effect, the golden rule—it all means the same thing: you get what you give. The people we like to classify as successful are all aware of universal law and operate by universal law. Being selfless is a universal law.

As the golden rule states in the Amplified Bible, "Whatever you desire that others would do to and for you, even so do also to and for them."[2] Therefore, if we want people to give us their best, we should give them our best. Please do not make the argument that millionaires and billionaires can give because they have time and money to give. We spoke on that in the last section called "Excuses." You can do a study on those who are considered to be financially successful, and you'll see that before they made their first million, they gave something to get there.

I'm not talking about those with what we call "old money," I am referring to those who have come from the bottom. The result of their success is based on the fact that they are using and sharing their time, talents, gifts, and treasures.

They have a service-first attitude, and because they have a service-first attitude, they have built businesses and empires based on service. Few people in America can say they have never used a personal computer, which is why Bill Gates is so wealthy. He serves millions. When we serve, we are giving of ourselves. Now we see why sharing was forced into our minds as children. It's natural, and it's beneficial. So give, serve, and lose the weight.

Unforgiveness

This section is a hard one, so I will do my best to prove to you that unforgiveness will hinder your progress. I know we don't like to hear the word *forgive*, especially when someone has done something to us that seems to be unforgivable. Unforgiveness is another rapidly spreading malignancy that will multiply at a moment's notice. It is another so-called friend who comes to the rescue when we are hurt. However, unforgiveness is another impersonator pretending to be something that it isn't, and that is our friend.

Oftentimes, we look at life as if it should be lenient toward us. We think to ourselves, *I'm not a bad person*, but we do not forgive the person who has wronged us. Life isn't biased to anyone, though it may seem that way. Life doesn't offer chains of bondage and barriers; people do. So why do we think we should be forgiven if we don't forgive?

As we already know, we live in a world of cause and effect. Unforgiveness sends a ripple into the universe, and though unseen, it makes an impact. It goes against everything that is natural and everything that is lawful. If we become unforgiving, we block the flow of energy and cause an imbalance. Sometimes, that block of energy and the imbalance can be felt and seen in our bodies in the form of cancer if our unforgiveness is allowed to metastasize into physical form. To be forgiving and to be trusting are two different things.

> Unforgiveness sends a ripple into the universe, and though unseen, it makes an impact.

A person who has wronged us has, of course, lost our confidence. So gaining our confidence back will be extremely difficult, though possible. However, forgiveness has nothing to do with confidence and everything to do with our rights. Forgiveness is giving up our right to treat people the same way they treated us. To forgive is to be the person in the forefront giving reconciliation before the other party does so.

Unforgiveness is taking away or undoing the other party's pretty bow of reconciliation. If you can imagine someone handing you a present in sincerity, and you untie the bow and drop the gift on the ground, you may be able to see that unforgiveness looks a little childish. Forgiveness is purely made by choice, so people who say they cannot forgive another person aren't being true to themselves. They can forgive and never associate with the person again; the one thing they don't want to do is clog up their flow of blessings with unforgiveness.

Being unforgiving will cause us to sacrifice energy we need on our way to success. We need all the energy that we can muster to travel the road of success. Unforgiveness is petty and will throw our lives off balance. So let's make the choice today to forgive those who have wronged us and lose the weight.

Worry

Worry cannot add a single hour to your life; conversely, it can take away from your life. Worry is an unhealthy habit that will and can diminish health. It is like sandpaper; over time, it wears us down. When we worry, we become anxious about a certain aspect of our lives. This anxiety will seriously affect us over time. We develop worry when we get ourselves into situations that we feel we have no control over.

Sometimes, worry comes without our doing. It may come as a sickness, or it may come by calamity. I remember when I played football in college, my head coach would always say, "Whatever is in your sphere of control is your responsibility to control, but if it is outside of your control, let God deal with it." I know that this is easier said than done, and it definitely doesn't mean to act as if there is nothing to worry about. Pretending that the situation isn't there will not cause it to disappear.

Our coach would then go on to give examples. He would say, "The forecast is saying there may be a chance for rain all week. Well, we can't control that, but what we can control is how we practice in the rain." It comes to a point where we have to make the decision whether we will work through the rain or idly sit by until it stops raining. We can be mindful of our situations while working through our circumstances with diligent labor until we see the sun peer from behind the clouds. Worry can appear on many different levels.

We can worry about waking up on time or how we're going to pay our bills. Some things we have control over, like the way we spend our money, and then other things we don't have control over, like losing our income stream. The things that we should give our undivided attention to are the things that we can influence by means of our control. If we can take care of our part, be thankful, because God will take care of the rest. We eliminate worry by diligently working and taking care of what we have control over. By doing this, we can assure ourselves every night that we gave it our best. Everyone should be able to live with their best effort. That being said, let's drop the pounds of worry and be healthy. Lose the weight.

Noise

You probably didn't realize this, but noise can potentially add on pounds also. In our society, noise is everywhere. We are lucky if the technology in our houses isn't making some form of noise at night as we sleep. The more mechanisms we build, the noisier our planet becomes. If we study some of the great thinkers of the past, we will find that they often sought solitude.

It's no surprise that they seemed to be much smarter. King David sought solitude to pray. Gandhi sought solitude to meditate. Even Isaac Newton was in a place of solitude underneath an apple tree when he conceived of an idea regarding the workings of gravity. They say silence is golden, and it truly is indeed. From silence, some of the world's best ideas, inventions, and innovations have come about. I truly believe that this tried, tested, and proved technique is the way to finding the next best idea in this era of producing change agents.

> From silence, some of the world's best ideas, inventions, and innovations have come about.

We must pull ourselves away from the computer, from the television, and even from that book in order to seek solitude and silence. In our society, solitude and silence are a joke. I have often wondered why the ancients and the great thinkers seemed so much smarter than those born after them. I came to the conclusion that it is a matter of silence. I believe that nothing is new under the sun; therefore, we have the brain capacity to think just as the ancients and great thinkers, but there is one thing hindering us, and that thing is noise.

Every day, million-dollar ideas are lurking in the dark waiting for someone to come to the realization that they're there. The one major negative proponent to this realization is in the form of competition with noise. These time-changing ideas compete with television, family, friends, and even our own scattered thoughts. Train yourself to adopt a life with time for daily seclusion and silence, and lose the weight of an abundance of noise distracters. Drop the weight.

Exercise

Step on my scale.

Losing unhealthy mental weight is essential to living mentally healthy.

What the world needs today is change and people who are mentally fit to bring that change.

1. First, identify your mental weight. Can you stand to lose some pounds? If so, what kind of weight do you need to lose? (For example, fear, doubt, indifference).
2. Identify how your weight has kept you back. Physically, extra weight places stress on the joints of the body, which causes pain. How has being mentally overweight caused you pain? By doing this, you can use your cause as a motivator when working to drop the weight.
3. What steps will you take to lose your weight? Have a well-written plan.

4. What are your expectations? When do you plan to be free from the added weight?

5. How will you implement the solutions given? Remember, in this case, awareness and honesty are the first steps to losing weight.

6. Go through the chapter again, and see how each trait can have an adverse affect on your life. Realize that if it affects your life, it affects others' as well.

Station 5—
Mental Strength: Bench-Press Your Problems

"To become mentally strong, one must hold in mind the weights of life by focus and concentration in an attempt to change the problems and stimulate the growth of the mind."

Mental strength is a very impressive quality to have. In it are all the characteristics of becoming a successful person. Across the globe, mental strength isn't very prevalent, but mental weakness is. Therefore, we must train ourselves to improve the strength of our mentality. It's very important for us to develop a habitual way of thinking that will push us until we're successful in our endeavors. The entirety of this book would mean nothing and have no effect on a person's life without the faculty of mental strength to implement the wisdom contained herewith. What are ways in which we can develop our strength mentally?

Stop Running

Don't run away or avoid problems; instead, take them head-on. A warrior's mentality is developed when a course of action isn't diverted, but when the decision is to take steps directly toward the problem or thing that is causing fear. All United States Marines know of the confidence course, where there are many seemingly impossible and fearful obstacles to cross. They are trained to take action and go straight forward to the problem. They attack the fear. They attack the difficulty.

To cause them to be a bit more zealous in attacking this course, they are paired up with a fellow recruit and are made to compete. The best way to attack problems and fear is to make it a game. Compete against yourself. If you're a salesman or saleswoman, compete alongside yourself, and when your mind is telling you, "That's enough. We don't want to hear anymore no's for the day," just collect your thoughts as a team would huddle up and say,

> The best way to attack problems and fear is to make it a game.

"Guys, we are not going to quit today. We have to get more; we have to do more. Who cares if we get twenty more no-thank-you's? We are going to keep asking so that even if we aren't as successful as we wanted to be, we'll know at the end of the day that we tried, and over and above our best is all we can give. Break!"

This may sound absurd, and you may not have to be as theatrical, but you must compete with yourself. Just like in the gym, do one more rep; do one extra minute on the bike; run one more mile. What I've found out as a personal trainer and as an athlete is that one more is all it takes to be better than the last. If we take this mind-set and do it every time, we will add on to what we did last.

So if we ran two miles one day, we'll do one more the next day, and one more the next day or week or month, all depending on our rate of progress. Progress will happen after consistent and conscious effort. Don't let yourself down. Most successful people feel guilty when they cheat themselves; therefore, they try not to do anything halfheartedly.

Don't cheat yourself. No one likes a cheater, and you'll find out quickly that you won't like yourself if you cheat. So get going in the correct direction and attack the problem. Build your mental strength.

Read and Learn New Words

Reading is a lost art in this day because of the ability of technology to hold our attention for an extended period of time. Reading is still paramount to the development of the brain and mind. Of course, if you are reading this book, you understand and appreciate this art. Many of the greats, from Mark Twain to Jim Rohn, understood the significance of knowing words and reading books. In essence, every person walking on the face of this earth is nothing more than a vessel that carries a spiritual equivalent to the manifestations in his or her life.

Essentially, we're all made up of a collection of ideas. Whatever ideas we carry are going to manifest in our lives. A collection of ideas is nothing more than a collection of words. So then, words are the building blocks to character. Words are used to shape and form. This is quite

> Essentially, we're all made up of a collection of ideas.

fascinating. Words have a spiritual quality to them that shapes the vessel in which they reside. The great men and women from past and present understood this, and they allowed only words that would cause them to become stronger mentally. Learn new words or use common words that will not only uplift you but also uplift the next person. When we uplift a neighbor, we are uplifted ourselves. In fact, it's easier to be uplifted by uplifting someone else than by merely focusing on ourselves.

Be Consistent

Find something in your life and stick to it. Become consistent with it. If it's a workout regimen, or reading one book a week, or giving five people a day a kind word, stick to it and don't back away from it.

You'll be amazed at how much this exercise will increase your focus and decision-making ability. You won't leave things to chance; you'll actually think of a solution. It may just be me but I have a theory. It seems that the people who take the time to make up the bed in the morning are the people who take the time to make up their minds in the morning.

Meaning what? Meaning that in their consistency of making up their beds, they are more likely to decide the actions of their day before they leave the house. As I said, this is only theory. Consistency builds mental strength because it causes a person to use the brain faculty to stay in routine. A routine becomes easier as it is performed, but it still takes mental effort to get it done. Most people walk around with a loose mind, not thinking much on anything constructive. They are in need of a toning up of their minds to lose the flabbiness that they have.

View Your World Objectively

Many of us tend to view our world the way we think it should be instead of how it really is. Now, I am not saying that we shouldn't hope for better, but delusion isn't a cure. When hoping for anything, there must be action to manifest that thing. No one who hopes to lose weight and doesn't take the steps necessary to lose the weight will succeed. Delusion is not our friend. The idea is to see and notice that the problem does exist.

We can't wish things away; we must work them away—meaning, faith without a little work is pointless. The only way to pinpoint the problem is to view the problem objectively for what it really is. Then we can view it the way we have decided it should be by believing and working, but this is only after objective circumspection.

Stepping into the Gym of Life

Every day we wake up, even before placing one foot out of bed, we mentally set foot inside of the *life gym*. The life gym is life itself. It's a privilege to be able to swipe our card each morning, verifying that our membership is still valid and we still have some work to do. Some gym memberships expire through the night, which is very unfortunate; therefore, each morning, when our eyes open, we should be ready to go to work. To be successful in a real gym, the best thing to do is to set our minds on improving and having a good workout, because otherwise, we're just wasting our money.

An efficient workout is a workout that is planned out in advance. Jumping from machine to machine isn't the best way to work out. This is a sure way to become indecisive. The same is true for our lives; become mentally strong by planning out your day so that indecision won't have room to grow. A good workout is one that empowers you in the end.

A good life workout in a day's work is one that will also empower you. Give it your all. Go over and above what you're asked to do; whether you are employed or self-employed, do more than is asked of you. This shapes and tones your mind and will have others asking you what you're doing to be so positive and mentally fit. If people spoke in this manner, they would say, "Wow, your mind looks terrific! You have so much more tone and more definition (clarity). Now I'm inspired to work out my mind too." Life is only hard because every day we wake up, it's there staring us in the face, and it's up to us to decide whether to improve or just to coast through. Build mental strength by using every opportunity in the gym to get better.

Don't Walk Past the Weights

When in the life gym, do you walk past the weights, or do you work with them? Do you take something that is trying to weigh you down and lift it up in mind? When we take a mental weight (i.e., bills, relationships, misfortunes, job) and hold it in our minds, we are exercising our minds to become stronger, not by stressing and being anxious, but by focusing on the issue with intensity and discernment. Most of us will decide either to walk by the weights or to lift them one time and put them back on the rack.

In order to build muscle, we need to perform repetitions so that our muscles can adapt. When solving problems, we cannot focus on them only a few times and move on to something else; we must sit there in our chairs and scrutinize the problem until it hurts. Once again, this isn't done in a stressful state but in a state that is calling for critical thinking. We can't use the abdominal roller for one minute and plop back down on the couch hoping to see results, nor can we muse over our bills for a few minutes and then float off into dreamland thinking that the problem is solved.

Can you remember how your muscles felt after a good workout? They felt sore and fatigued, right? Sometimes in our quest to lift up a problem in order to solve it, we can become mentally fatigued. This is when we take a break and come back to it later. If you've experienced this before, you have probably realized that when you come back to it, you're better able to think and come up with solutions.

Just in that short amount of time, your mind recovered from the stress placed on it. Amazing! Back in college, I learned a way to study for my finals that worked for me each time. I would go over my notes by trying to incorporate every sense I could. I would read aloud and walk around the room. I would even try to vividly imagine what I was reading, but this wasn't the secret to my success.

The secret was in that I studied and rehearsed the information over and over again until it felt like I couldn't think anymore, and I continued until I was very sleepy. After this session of repetition upon repetition, I would then immediately, without doing anything else, fall asleep. The next morning, when going over my notes, I saw that memorizing the information wasn't as hard as it had been the night before. By the morning, I had gained mental muscle and was able to memorize (lift) the material (weight) more easily than before.

Recover from Stress

Muscle is gained when pressure or force is applied to it, which then causes microtears. The muscle in these microtears grows back bigger and stronger if it is given the proper ingredients, such as protein and rest. Every now and again, we'll succumb to mental stress, even if just for a moment. We have so many things applying force to our minds that microtears in our mental makeup are a result. To grow bigger and stronger mentally is to nourish these microtears back to good health by proper nutrition and adequate rest. Nutrition includes positive mind food, which is primarily faith and belief. Faith is the building block of a strong mind. Just as a muscle needs protein to grow, our minds need faith to grow. Without faith, a strong mind isn't possible. A strong mind is a result of believing in something wholeheartedly.

Consume faith daily. The Bible says that solving huge problems only requires a small amount of faith. The faith we need is insignificantly small. This sounds very simple, but if it was, everyone would be doing it. A large group of people struggle with having an insignificantly small amount faith that has enough power to move any problem in their lives up to the size of what seems like a mountain. The problem with most people is that they neutralize their small faith by mixing it with doubt. In order for faith to work, it cannot be diluted with doubt; it loses its potency. Be sure to train your mind daily, but also be sure to consume faith daily to counteract the minor mental microtears.

Stay Flexible

It's been reported that stretching on your off days can sustain your strength level until you go back to the gym to get stronger. Once you've done the work to build up a muscle group, experts say the next best thing to do when not working out is to stretch. How can we stretch mentally? We went over this in a previous chapter. We have to take a look at the things that we're using to build our minds.

Is it being more mentally aware of our surroundings or more mentally sensitive to other people's feelings, or is it overcoming our fears? On our off periods (maybe at night or on weekends), we must stretch in order to maintain the strength. In this instance, stretching is nothing more than just mentally going over what we have improved for that day or week. Did we improve our awareness, did we improve our sensitivity, or did we take steps to conquering our fears? If so, we have gained strength. Reinforce the strength built by musing over the workout. At night, think about and ponder your courage. Keep a journal so that pondering over your accomplishments will be easier to follow. And as you ponder think even bigger. What will you do next time that will trump your success today? Remember, next time, perform one more rep. In this way, we are stretching our belief system and maintaining our strength until we are able to go back out and actually put in more work.

Exercise

Pick up the weight of life and lift it.

Mental strength is a must for all who desire to improve their lives.

1. Reading is still essential. Each day, read books that will offer you more knowledge and help you think to a greater capacity. Learn new words. Use uplifting words to uplift yourself and someone else.
2. Attack your fear head-on. Don't wait and think about it. Do it now!
3. Become the person who loves the gym. Love life, and use

the issues, circumstances, and problems of life to make you better. Lift up the weight and focus on improvement.

4. Don't worry about what you can't control. Anxiety is not good for your health. Focus on and give your attention only to things you can control. Leave the rest to God.

5. At the end of your day, right before you go on break (sleep), ponder your accomplishments. What did you do well today? What could you have improved on? Did you smile at someone today? Did you offer to help someone else? Think on these things, and desire to outdo yourself the next day.

Station 6—Mental Endurance: Breathe Inspiration to Sustain Life and Health

"Resuscitating a breathless person and resuscitating a breathless dream are two things everyone should learn how to do."

A strong cardiovascular system is significant to good health. In the term *cardiovascular*, we are referring to the ability of the heart to pump blood throughout our body. When our body is highly sufficient in delivering the needed oxygen to the working muscles via the lungs, heart, and blood vessels, we deem this cardiovascular endurance. At the root of this definition is the importance of having a strong cardiovascular system and muscular endurance, which is what allows the muscle to do repeated work without fatigue.

You may be wondering how this relates to mental endurance. The significance of mental endurance is just as important as physical endurance in that our mind's can become fatigued after continuous work in well doing. Well doing is any action that you perform to better your life, such as doing more than what's asked of you, sticking to a good habit you've formed, reading something inspirational each day, being humble, or being of good cheer when everything around you says to feel the opposite. Most importantly, however, well doing is any action to help improve someone else's life. Taking from what we know of the process of the cardiovascular system, when we draw a parallel to that of the mind we can conclude that in order to develop mental endurance one must develop a strong mental heart, mental lungs, and enrich the mental blood system. This may sound confusing now, but as we go on I'll explain what all of this means. Even now you can think on these illustrations and parallels for yourself and see if you can understand the similarities.

We'll go back to what we previously mentioned on the subject of the mental heart. We only briefly touched on a few points, mainly on how to build a heart. We will summarize that information briefly, but our focus will be on other aspects of the mental heart and how important it is to have a healthy mental heart.

Of course, we saw that a mental heart is composed of our truths and nothing but our truths mixed with strong emotion. Therefore, truth to the mental heart is the equivalent of blood to the physical heart and emotion is similar to ventricular

> Therefore, truth to the mental heart is the equivalent of blood to the physical heart and emotion is similar to ventricular contractions.

contractions. Truth is the source of life to the mental heart, and without it circulating in and through our mental heart, the vitality of our belief-system will expire. It's impossible to have a heart without strong emotion attached to it. Emotion is what keeps your truths flowing through your belief-system, meaning that emotion is what keeps your beliefs vibrant.

This is why it's usually not wise to discuss religion, politics, and finances with a complete stranger. The two individuals are oblivious in knowing what the other believes concerning any of the categories above. And when there is a difference in belief between the two, it's possible that they may become emotional and contentious. This emotion is surfaced because when a person's beliefs are confronted, emotion is what keeps their beliefs vibrant and alive. They refuse to let their beliefs die so they use emotion as a way of pumping inspiration (facts reinforcing their belief) to their mental heart to sustain the system. The greater the emotion the greater the pump. This is similar to a person performing physical exercise where the body is under stress to pump an increased amount of blood to the rest of the body. This is why ventricular contractions, which pump blood through the heart, is similar to emotion which pumps truth through the mental heart. Therefore, we see here in a real life situation how emotion sustains the flow of our beliefs.

I mention the expression of truth as being the blood to the mental heart, but this truth isn't necessarily absolute truth, it's what you believe to be true which can ultimately be false or faulty. If this then is the case we must be diligent in what way we construct our hearts. Since the occupation of a heart is to house our personal truths, it will cost us if we construct a heart that cannot withstand the tests and trials of life. The value in taking the time to construct a sturdy heart surmounts the low cost of awareness and knowledge it takes to build it. We mustn't build a heart that is based on sand, but rather one whose foundation is on rock. This rock is absolute truth. Now, I understand that when dealing with people, our hearts are not able to have a foundation of absolute truth concerning them, but we can build the heart concerning that person on the absolute truth foundation of love. Love never fails, even when it seems as if it does. Love doesn't fail; people fail.

Be Imitators

The tool of the intellect isn't short of responsibility, as it has the toughest job. It is up to our mind to decide what we will become. If this is the case, it would be wise to feed our minds with the right substances and observe successful people. Put yourself around success, whether it is a successful person or a successful environment. Do not follow after the patterns of the unsuccessful but after the patterns of the successful.

Follow after the patterns of those individuals who have proved to have a successful life. This starts at the level of thought. Ask this question: what kind of mind did these people have? I use the past tense here, but I'm also referring to those successful people who are still living. You should gain the same state of mind that they have and adopt it so that you can also have a winning attitude.

We want our minds to be the team captain and great leaders. Being an imitator is not as bad as some try to make it seem. As the adage goes: if it's not broken, don't fix it. For a while now, successful people have preached upon the fact that anyone who wants to be successful should follow the habits of other successful people. Just as they are followers of success and imitators of those who mentored them, we should also be imitators and followers of their success principles.

Granted, we're all unique and should be our own person; what I mean by imitating is following their system. What did they do to reach their level of success? How did they think? What did they read? In order for all of this to happen, we must make a conscious decision that we will learn from these people.

We must make up our minds to be imitators of those who have made an awesome life for themselves. We must guard our minds from all things that will hinder our dreams and goals. We must bring every thought to the submission of truth, and that truth is what we are striving for. If that thought doesn't line up with where we want to go in life, it must be cast down, snatched out of the sky, and destroyed. Success begins in and with the mind.

This isn't something that is clandestine and concealed only for a special elite group. This knowledge and wisdom is for all who will listen and become a student of its truths. Remember, whatever we allow to dwell in our minds, we will eventually become by default and even by program. We must stand guard at the gate of our minds and not allow the agents of sabotage to enter the place in our minds where we truly believe and feel strongly about any given thing; we must be very conscious of what we allow to lodge at the front gate.

Mental Terrorism

We must guard that place with all assiduousness, because this place is where life is constructed and springs to the surface. The guard at the front gate is our conscious mind. Our conscious mind is the guard who is aware of who is roaming past our gate. The gate is to our heart and subconscious mind. We don't allow everything to enter through this gate, because not everything is in our best interest. This is likened to an embassy in a foreign country. Not everyone who comes to the gate of the embassy will be allowed in because they may not be authorized to enter. The same is true for us. This world is not our home, but is foreign land. We're ambassadors in this land we call earth. We find protection behind the gate in the embassy palace. Here, we are in connection with the motherland and or President, and in this case the president is God. We meet God in our heart. Therefore, nothing shall pass our gate that is not authorized to enter.

Much sabotage can and will happen if we fail to guard this gate. The world in which we live has seen an increase in terrorism, but terrorism is as ancient as man and woman. The original form of terrorism is thought. We have thoughts that will assimilate to our good thoughts, but to a man, the way may seem right when there is destruction thereof. There are thoughts of fear that seem to be in our best interest, which will come and stand at the gate.

This fear may suggest, "You may not want to take this particular risk."

Sometimes we say, "You know what? You're right!" We allow this perpetrator to enter our palace, but we don't realize that once it enters, it'll cause chaos and create havoc. Then when we want to do something that will improve our lives, there isn't enough harmony and order within ourselves to carry it out. Fear has sent us back to the dark ages, when we didn't have the knowledge that we could do whatever we placed our minds to. Therefore, it is paramount to distinguish friend from foe.

Just as with people, we cannot be trusting of all of our thoughts. We must take *all* of the thoughts that roam through our minds captive. We must apprehend them and question their allegiance. We must sit these thoughts in a wooden chair in an empty room with only one bright light shining down on their faces. Place the spotlight on these thoughts and interrogate them (figuratively speaking).

We must bring our thoughts into captivity and bring them to the submission of our dreams, goals, and plans for our lives. We must question these thoughts along the lines of loyalty to our goals, dreams, visions, and aspirations. Some thoughts seem to mean well, but meaning well doesn't help the cause. We should ask questions like: Why are you here? What is your motive? Will you help us go forward? What is your underlying action? Who are you really working for? Will you hinder performance, or will you push performance along? This may seem absurd, but thinking about what you're thinking about isn't new.

Controlling one's thoughts has been a staple of success for thousands of years!

Any thought that will try to usurp power from the true laws of God must be put down immediately, without hesitation. If we ever have a thought that says it is better to receive than to give, it's not in our best interest, and it

> Any thought that will try to usurp power from the laws of God must be put down immediately, without hesitation.

must be put down. If we have a thought that says we don't need to have love for all, it must be put down immediately. By no means should you allow this thought to carry its sabotage and destruction into your palace. Maintain the peace and the order in your heart.

If you're visual, you're probably visualizing a military form of inner government that keeps guard and protects, and it's just that: a military. The soldiers consist of a well-disciplined and well-trained unit that knows how to fight and protect the palace. These soldiers have names like courage, confidence, love, persistence, excellence, peace, self-control, discipline, and integrity, among others. This is a mighty fighting unit, and there is strength in numbers. This fighting unit will fight for us and is in our best interest, but they must be trained. We are the drill instructors, but God is the Master Instructor.

He is the one who will place us in situations that will cause us to rise to another level. He will train these soldiers to make them sufficient in battle. They have to be trained to be diligent and orderly. They must be trained to be the first on the scene, and they must be trained never to sleep but to stand and keep guard, protecting our palace. And the only weapon that they fight with is the weapon of truth.

Nothing can defeat and have victory over this high-tech weapon. Truth blasts anything unlike it to smithereens. Universal truths are the laws of God, and nothing can stand against them. So we must be mindful to build up our army and train them well to keep us safe and protect our palace from those who would like to destroy us. Train these soldiers in the grueling process of recognizing truth, and nothing that means us harm will have prosperity over us. We will always and forever be conquerors and victorious.

Watch What You Put on Film

If I can relate back to my years of playing football in college, I remember our head coach would always tell us to be aware of what we were putting on film. In football, there are meetings in which the team will sit in an auditorium-like room and view themselves from a previously recorded practice or game. This is done to learn from mistakes or from things done well. You may or may not know this, but football isn't just about running into one another; the physicality of football is just the half of it. The game of football, believe it or not, is a well-thought-out, fast-paced game.

Players from the college ranks to the professional ranks and even some high school teams watch film to get a gauge on the tendencies of their opponent. We were taught to watch anything, such as if a particular player leans to the right or to the left on certain plays and where a player looks, or what stance a player takes on particular plays to know when the ball is going to be passed or run. We tried to find anything that would give us the edge. However, the same is true for everyone else. If we were looking for tendencies, everyone else was looking for the same tendencies, so our coach would always say, "Watch what you put on film!" We should ask ourselves, "What am I putting on film?"

Mind

What are we putting on the film of our minds? What tendencies are we giving away? We have an opponent out there watching and studying our clues and giveaways to our weaknesses. Just as the objective of football is to find a weakness and attack that weakness so that the football can find its way into the end zone, the objective of our opponent is to find a possible way to win a one-on-one battle and enter our palace.

The opponent is none other than the perpetrators we have been discussing already. Fear knows your weakness, and it attacks that weak point. The thought of lack knows your weakness, and it attacks that weak point. Remember the saying "A chain is only as strong as its weakest link." What is your weakest link? Who on your team can't be trusted?

I believe the saying "Teamwork makes the dream work" is fitting here. Clearly, this is a game called life, and those who are the most prepared to play this game will be the victors. We can hear coaches of all sports voicing those confident words, "We will not be out prepared!" Do not let life out prepare you. Life has a considerable jump on us, so it is pretty learned in its occupation. We also must be learned in this occupation of life if we want to be successful and reap the benefits of the hard labor of preparation.

Will

Will is the guy of action and word. Remember when people used to say, "All I have is my word." This was before contracts, civil suits, and court cases. Well, you may not remember that, but you may have heard of the saying before. This saying is synonymous with the functions of our will.

Our will, will show up in our actions and our words. As a matter of fact, our will is our actions and our words. Quite simply, our will is what we will to happen. That sounds easy enough, right? The way that we will things in our lives is first by thinking them and then acting on them. This is where our will comes in.

Have you ever told a person before, "No, I will not do that"? Well, obviously, whatever that person was trying to get you to do was against what you were willing to do, but the point is that whatever they meant for you to do, you could only do by word or action. So they probably said, "Hey, I dare you to say this …" or "I dare you to do that …" Whatever it is that they dare you to do will always be aimed at your actions and words. Our will nowadays resembles our world. No one really keeps their word anymore.

You may be saying, "I keep my word," but if you told yourself you were going to eat healthily at the turn of the year and you failed to do so, you broke your word. You went against your will. What you were willing to do, you are no longer able. I believe that it's pandemic in regard to how easy it is for us to break our word. This is why our society is full of people who decide to do just whatever it is that they please because people don't have control over themselves anymore.

We just will do whatever it is we will (to) do. No control and no limits equal troubles ahead. We need to develop our willpower again. Just think about how our view of world health would be if people were able to say no to some things. What about the financial crisis and bailing out banks and the poor housing market in the millennium's first decade?

How different that might be if people were willing to both say no and keep their word. What are you willing to do? What are we willing to do together as a world? Willingness is the beginning of action. Who is willing to change for the better?

Who will say, "I will to change"? A will and testament isn't always for the day we die. A will and testament can also be for the time in which we are living. What are we willing to do? What service will we hand over and to which persons will we hand it? Service is the giving of ourselves. Service is the best gift we can give. What better gift can we give than ourselves? None. Service is the beginning of receiving. To what will we give testament? And once we give our word, will we keep it?

Will we, in ourselves, prove our words through our actions? Or will we be remembered for breaching word agreements? It's time for the people of this world to return to their morals and values, which once included doing something as small as keeping their word. A thought will always remain just a thought until it is buried in the courtyard of our hearts and allowed to germinate. Once we do that, our thoughts will cease to be only thoughts and germinate into action, and this is the fruit of all thought. The perpetuation of success in our lives begins when we give ourselves permission to be successful.

The way in which we give ourselves permission is when we will ourselves to go above what the world has to say about situations, such as the level of our schooling, the economy, our age, our race or ethnicity, or even our socioeconomic status. Our will has to grow in stature and wisdom as our minds grow. As we grow in confidence, we will cause ourselves to strive after more opportunities that this life brings.

Emotions

Emotions are like the worker bees of the entire operation. Worker bees work tirelessly for the rest of the hive. As the queen nests in the hive, the workers fly about and conduct daily business. Without the worker bees, the colony would cease to exist. There can be a CEO and there can be a manager, but if there aren't any workers, then production ceases.

It is the workers who carry along the plans of the top officials. Any company knows how valuable the workers are. No workers means no business. Our emotions should be trained to perform and operate in diligence. We never want to get to the point where we are controlled by our emotions, but we want to be in the position where we're in control of them.

As I said, emotions are nothing more than workers. Wherever the top officials are planning for the company to go, the emotion workers will work to get it there. Our emotions were never meant to go erratic, but to be channeled toward a definite purpose and

> Our emotions were never meant to go erratic but to be channeled toward a definite purpose and focus.

focus. However, most of us allow our emotions to be wasted by allowing them to run wherever they choose. It's more like an unattended day care.

If children are not watched with close supervision, they can and will get into a lot of trouble, and the same is true for our emotions. We have to supervise what we are feeling and especially what we are feeling strongly about. If we fail to monitor our emotions, it is possible that they will have an adverse effect on us. I say this because our emotions have a habit of ingraining patterns of behavior and memory into our subconscious mind, and we know that the subconscious mind is really the Big Kahuna. The subconscious mind (heart) holds a lot of clout, and everyone listens to it, including the conscious mind, the will, and the emotions.

It's like the mob boss, whom no one sees but everyone obeys, sitting in the back corner of a dark room smoking a cigar. Guard your emotions closely, since emotion has the ability to quicken your thoughts. There is a correlation between spirit, breath, and emotion, in that emotion allows our thoughts to live and breathe. Emotions breathe into the nostrils of our thoughts, and our thoughts become alive (spirit-filled). By breathing emotion into our thoughts, we become inspired.

The best way to become inspired is by word and by testimony. By reading this book, you are becoming inspired. You are becoming inspired to take the reins of your life, and you are giving breath and life to your dreams and goals. Listening to

> Emotion breathes into the nostrils of our thoughts, and our thoughts become alive.

the testimony of others who are successful is also a source of inspiration. We don't want to smother and asphyxiate our dreams by limiting their supply of inspiration (air).

Many worthy and attainable dreams are born overnight but often die because there is a lack of inspiration, which would allow them to breathe. We fail to read books and listen to success stories. Jim Rohn once said, "We put valuable things on the high shelf, so you can't get to them until you're qualified. If you want the things on the higher shelf, you've got to stand on the books you read." Books are a very important resource in helping people become successful. Books are like a form of exercise for the mind—a nice jog around the block.

Jogging opens up the lungs and allows oxygen to rush in and circulate through the bloodstream. Reading opens up the lungs of the mind and allows inspiration to flow and circulate through our mental heart and spirit. Sometimes, a testimony is similar to resuscitation. Sometimes, someone can give an account of their failures and successes, and that will be like the resuscitation of our goals and dreams, bringing them back to life and giving them another chance to live. So reading and hearing the life stories of others who have failed and have then succeeded will keep our dreams and goals alive and growing.

Made in His Image and Likeness

I will show how similar man and woman are to the image and likeness of God. The God of the Bible is identified also as the Trinity. The Trinity is recognized as three separate and distinct individuals who are still one and whole with no separation. This is tantamount to saying there is harmony and unity within the Holy Trinity, but it still does no justice in truly explaining the sovereignty and harmony of God. The Trinity consists of the Father God, Jesus Christ, and the Holy Spirit. We can see clear evidence that we are made in the image and likeness of God by observing the fact that the Father God is parallel to the mind, Jesus Christ is parallel to the will, and the Holy Spirit is parallel to the emotions.

To put it bluntly, the Trinity, in operation, is similar to our soul. Our soul is one entity, but it is three, just like the Holy Trinity. In the process of building the world and the universe, God only worked with principles of truth. He created nothing that didn't have truth in it. What that means to us is that God built His heart, so to speak, not like we, who are fairly biased, do, but by placing His heart in His work-actually quite literally.

What He built is what He truly believes. All that God created was solely based on how He truly felt. His creations are an expression of His feelings and thoughts. God, or the Trinity, worked together in unison to build and create, just as we must do within our soul to build and create. His material that He built and constructed with came from within Himself, and all of creation is based on how he truly feels about the heavens and the earth, how He felt about us and His angelic host, and how He felt about Himself. We can see that He felt magnificent by that for which He has built a heart.

One Accord

What happens when our tools aren't in accordance with one another? Our mind believes one thing, our will wants to do something different, and our emotions are feeling differently about what we believe and what we want to happen. Dysfunction and strife in the inner world will translate to dysfunction and strife in the outer world. We have to learn how to place our tools in accordance with one another. While this sounds like common sense, it really isn't. If this was common sense, success and prosperity would be more common in individual lives and as a result more prevalent in the world, but they aren't. We should take a lesson out of our music books.

Harmony is achieved when three notes are struck together at the same time making one chord—in one accord. *Harmony* is the key word that we are looking for. Harmony is the lubricant to a life filled with friction in the form of fear, hate, envy, jealousy, contention, and strife. If harmony is in the atmosphere, things work smoothly, but if there is discord in the atmosphere, the result is friction, and some things come to a screeching halt.

Therefore, we should not hope that success and abundance can be achieved if we have discord in our soul. Our mind, our will, and our emotions must work together toward a common goal. This is the magic of the number three. Harmony is found in three, and where there is harmony, there is progress.

Flow of Truth

It is imperative that we have enough truth flowing through our hearts if we expect this truth to be the life source of our dreams. Our hearts play a vital role in giving life to our visions and dreams. If we do not truly believe that we can have that thing that we are hoping for, it will not come to fruition. Absolute belief is the beginning of claiming the things that we truly believe we can have. If we have absolute belief, that is evidence of the things that we do not see physically as being possible to accomplish.

Just as our physical hearts are in continuous rhythm, beating and pumping blood throughout our bodies, replenishing our bodies with oxygen-rich blood, our mental hearts are continuously pulsating truth through our beings via emotion. This is why affirmations are so powerful. Affirmations are to the mind what air is to the body. We must affirm what we believe constantly to supply and reinforce our personal truth. And an active affirmation is like exercise. Exercise is great because it requires us to take in a greater amount of oxygen than we normally would.

This translates into oxygen-rich blood. We should relate this to exercising our affirmations daily. Sitting down for a number of minutes a day and exercising with our affirmations will increase the richness of our belief. Notice that I said sitting down and reciting our affirmations is like exercising. We don't exercise all day, but we do breathe all day. Similarly, all we need is a few minutes each day to exercise our affirmations by intense focus, but we are obliged to constantly repeat and rep our affirmations, by thought, word, and action. This is breathing.

Breathe Heavily

If you haven't noticed yet—which I believe would be impossible, but if you haven't noticed—I take the physical component of our bodies and draw a parallel to help us better understand the mind. Here, I would like to compare another similarity concerning the respiratory systems of both the body and the mind. We know that once the body is involved in strenuous activity that affects the cardiovascular system, the brain sends out a signal that says, *"We need more air!"* When the signal goes out, we begin to breathe heavily, forcing more air into our lungs. If we still aren't getting enough air, our brains scream out, *"The system is failing! More air! More air!"* Then we breathe even more heavily, forcing even more air into our lungs. If we fail to keep up with the demand, all operations shut down and we black out.

Our brains command in earnest, *"Shut down all engines now! Maybe we can save the ship!"* I'm giving this illustration because I would like to present my parallel of this bodily function to the mental function. As we go through life, it can get awfully difficult. Sometimes, we even go through days when we struggle to get out of bed and embark on the day because of fear or dread of what the day holds. This is a miserable way to live.

We may get into a state of having our breath taken away, or we may be waiting for that moment when we can exhale, but sometimes in life, those moments don't come fast enough. When life gets hard and strenuous and our minds are running and racing, we become mentally out of breath. Weary and tired, all we want is for it to end. We would just like a moment to stop and catch our breath. In this instance, our mind is screaming for more *air*, but often we either ignore its demands or we don't comprehend what it's calling for.

In moments like these, we need more air, and the equivalent to that is inspiration. Inspiration keeps us lively. It keeps us enthused and holds our dreams, goals, and visions close and in view. I recently heard this saying, "Are you living, or are you just existing?" The living that this person was referring to was the living that would allow people

> Inspiration is the act of inhalation (of a substance) that generates power to move the intellect and emotions.

to dream big, plan out their paths, and attack the plan, not become stagnant in life like so many of us do.

I find *inspiration* to be a special word worth studying with careful consideration. *Webster's New Explorer Dictionary* defines *inspiration* as inhalation or the act or power of moving the intellect or emotions.[3] When we take these two definitions and think about the mind, we can conclude that inspiration is the act of inhalation (of a substance) that generates power to move the intellect and emotions.

I believe this is a powerful description. What substance can be drawn in to cause a movement of our intellect and emotions? Well, for one, a book like this or any other book that encourages the reader to strive and reach for the best or any audio material that encourages the same thing, but most important, we can draw from the stored information that we have locked away in our brains—things that we have read and heard and even circumstances and situations that we've gone through and have overcome. I once worked closely beside a friend who was inspired by what he believed he could do.

He told me a story about the struggles and trials he had faced and overcame by perseverance. In his professional football career, he was a draftee in a late round. His first season was good, but then he suffered an injury. The team later released him from his contract, and he was out of work, injured, and struggling to make it financially. Even though he was injured, his will was hurt more than anything else.

Rock bottom he did hit, but then, as he explained, he made up his mind that he was going to make a comeback. Since he didn't have much money, he couldn't buy training equipment, such as cones, so he borrowed old pairs of shoes and placed them strategically out in the field to practice his cuts and agility. How determined must he have been to use shoes as cones? It paid off, because he was signed by another team and had a great career, becoming team captain on his last professional team. He has since retired, and now has a very successful business. I know that he has kept those trying times with him so that he can pull from and be inspired by them.

We can probably think of a time in our lives when we overcame and achieved when the odds were against us. If that's not a reality, there are plenty of success stories out there that we can draw from to generate power through someone else's testimony and move our intellect and emotions. Remember, it is our emotions that drive us and keep us going after the dream. When our chips are down and our minds are begging for inspiration to continue, all we need to do is pull from a source that will encourage us to continue trucking. Once this habit is formed, nothing will by any means stop us.

We will find new means by which to accomplish our goals. This is where the intellect comes into play. Inspiration improves the intellect, because once we say, "I will not be caught breathless!" and continue to inspire ourselves, our minds will find a way to reach our desired destiny. Consider this point: depending on the stress level, depending on how fast we are running or exerting energy, our body will always call for a greater amount of air, and so it is also with our minds. The harder life gets, the more stressful it becomes, and the more discouraging the issues we face, the more our minds will call for a greater amount of inspiration, which we will need to pull in to sustain the life of our dreams.

Asthma, the Dream Snatcher

During my years in elementary school, I developed a mild case of asthma. Thank God I have since grown out of it. Asthma is a disease of the respiratory system, sometimes caused by allergies, with symptoms including coughing, sudden difficulty in breathing, and a tight feeling in the chest. I remember having to go into the clinic after recess to take a few puffs from my asthma pump because I was wheezing, but I never endured a life-threatening situation. I disliked asthma because my teachers were extra careful, watching over me for any flare-ups.

As I said, my asthma was a mild case, but they couldn't take any chances. I'm sure that there are many children and adults out there who have serious cases of asthma who can't do much out of fear of an episode. I currently deal with what some may call seasonal allergies. However, my allergies aren't seasonal; they can spring up whenever. In some cases, victims' allergies are as enduring and annoying as asthma. From sneezing to headaches, it all takes a toll on the lives of these people, but is it possible for all people to suffer from a mental form of asthma?

Of course, those who suffer from a natural form of asthma are a disproportionately smaller group than those without, but those who have mental cases of asthma amount in the millions. As most cases of natural asthma are developed in childhood, so are mental cases of asthma. We learn so much in our adolescence, and oftentimes, this is the time when we develop who we are. We can develop a winning attitude or behavior or we can develop a losing attitude or behavior. Having a poor attitude restricts the flow of positive self-talk and affirmations (air).

It restricts our ability to inspire ourselves. Have you ever seen someone with a poor attitude being inspired? Seldom, right? This is a mental case of asthma, and it all begins with the way we behave, and the way we behave is based on the way we think. Psychologists say behavior is the way a person responds to a specific set of conditions.

We should ask ourselves this question: "How am I responding to my current condition?" If your current set of conditions are poor, examine your attitude to see if you think there is someone else to blame or if it's just the hand that life has dealt you. We can always make adjustments with the hand we have, but excuses never solve anything. What if you have everything? Do you assume the role of being better than those who do not? Or do you consider yourself to be fortunate? What if you're in the middle, where you don't have it all but you have enough, pretty much like I was growing up? Are you appreciative of what you have, or are you constantly craving more? We should be honest with ourselves in answering these questions, because it will say plenty about our current attitude. Our attitudes determine how high we go, and our behavior determines where we go.

However, a large part of both are formed in our childhood. We get a gauge early on in life about how high we can go and where we can go. Unfortunately, this may be a result of our environment, but at this time, if we have a bad attitude or unruly behavior, it is something that we can change. It is never too late for progress, and it's never too late to treat mental asthma. If we can't breathe and be inspired, living will be difficult in the context of living our dreams.

Breathing is a two-way process. We breathe in, and then we breathe out. The diaphragm is the muscle responsible for pulling in and pushing out air. It is a curved muscular membrane below the rib cage. This is the muscle that singers and actors and actresses are trained to build up, because the diaphragm controls the flow of air. When we breathe in, we pull in fresh oxygen, and this oxygen travels throughout our bodies via our blood vessels. As this fresh oxygen travels, it becomes toxic to our bodies and converts to carbon dioxide.

This is why our bodies force out carbon dioxide. As stated earlier, inspiration is the act of breathing in fresh air in the form of affirmations, inspiring books, inspiring audio, or from our own memory banks. As we travel through life and as we acquire inspiration from different sources, the world of disappointment, doubt, and fear takes its toll on our supply of positive thinking; therefore, sometimes the inspiration that once was vibrant in us can and will be depleted. Just like the body pulls the oxygen from our blood in order that it may continue to function, the world pulls our inspiration from us in order that it may continue to function, because the world cannot function without fear. If the world can strip us of our faith and inspiration, then it can continue to act as the world, producing and striving in fear.

As long as we live in this world, we will not be able to escape this. Through exercise and practice, we may be able to convert fewer toxins, but nevertheless, the toxins will always be a part of our lives. Breathing starts with the diaphragm. In mental terms, our diaphragm is our ability to concentrate on pulling the right things in and squeezing all others out. When we concentrate intently on our affirmations and sources of information, we are pulling in fresh inspiration that will keep our dreams and goals alive and well.

The world takes its toll on our positive thinking and positive self-talk. When this happens our thinking becomes tainted and toxic, because of depletion. Therefore, we need to squeeze or push out the toxins. We

> We have to be able to concentrate on all of the other attributes of success in order for those success principles to work.

do this by contracting our minds in a way that would cause the toxins to be removed expediently from our system of thought. This is nothing more than concentration, closing our minds to negative, defeatist speech and thought and pushing out anything that may hinder us. Concentration is the secret to progress. We have to be able to concentrate on all of the other attributes of success in order for those success principles to work.

If we can focus our minds on what we want to accomplish day in and day out, we won't lose focus on the prize. Concentration is the focus of intellect and resources. The resources that we have pulled from and inspired ourselves with will come in handy at this point in time. This is the best time to take all of our resources and concentrate them toward one goal, and that is forcing out negativity by putting positivity in its place. This is the time to contract our minds in concentration, pulling on every bit of inspiration that we have retained and forcing out the things that would threaten our livelihood.

Exercise

Are you living a rich life, drawing on much inspiration, or are you asphyxiating?

1. What are the conditions of your heart? Is it strong enough to support your lifestyle? Are there any abnormal rhythmic patterns (indecisiveness, unbelief)? Identify your belief system. Is what you believe truly what you have taught your heart to believe? There is a difference.

2. Do you take care of your heart by exercising? Exercise with your affirmations daily. Sit down a number of minutes a day and focus intently on them. Reinforce what you believe. Build a strong and dynamic heart.

3. If we were to train in Denver where the air is thin, we would force our bodies to breathe deeply. Pretend each day that

your mind is training in Denver. Breathe deeply and inspire yourself daily.

4. Read inspirational material. Remind yourself daily of hardships that you have pulled through.

5. Listen to inspirational messages.

6. Work on your diaphragm to forcefully push out negativity. Concentrate on the best, and push out negative thoughts.

7. Practice controlled breathing. Be aware of what you allow to influence you.

Part 2

How to Get to Your Destiny

- Arriving
- Preparation
- Determination and Persistence
- Progress
- Good Stewardship
- Living

Station 7—
Arriving at Your Destination

"A man's gift maketh room for him, and bringeth him before great men" (Prov. 18:16, KJV).[4]

If destiny were a destination (which it is), purpose would be the reason to travel. Passion would be the road to get there, and preparedness would be the things we pack up to go. Sounds like the makings of a road trip to me. We have a place to go; we have a reason for going; we have the map to get there; and we're all packed up. Passion keeps us steady on the path to our destination, while purpose is the reason we are going. By finding our purpose in life and maintaining passion, we can meet our destiny.

This is a concise description of what life is intended to be. God has given us a reason for being here and has planned a destination for us to reach. The reason for being is usually to solve some problem presiding in the world. I know that some believe that they're insignificant and have no power to create change in this world, but all things start on a small level. Do not forsake humble beginnings. If we can work on doing the little things and focusing on making a change on our own level, then these changes will grow to something bigger. Just think if everyone had this mind-set what could get done.

Unfortunately, not everyone does have this mind-set. Many, instead, choose to compare their lives to those of the activist or the journalist or the author who is getting the most attention in changing things for the better. These individuals look at themselves and say, "Well, what am I good for?" We have to remember that the activist and the well-known journalist didn't start on a grand scale; they started small, probably trying to bring change to their households or neighborhoods or community centers. If you are trying to bring change for the betterment of others and not for selfish gain, God will give you a platform from which to speak. Just remember that one of your reasons for existing is to solve a problem. You are here to be the solution to a problem. You must add value to the world and not take away the value that others before you have instituted.

Just like a homeowners' association, you should do what it takes to keep up the property value of your neighborhood because you have a vested interest. The property which I am alluding to here is the world we live in. We all share the same planet, so why not do our part to add value to our property? It starts with passion. This is why God has given us motivational gifts; our gifts will line up with our passions.

There is one important factor that we should take into consideration here. We know the saying, "If you fail to plan, you plan to fail." Preparation is of top concern and importance. If we prepare, the opportunity will present itself. The other two aspects, purpose and passion, we do not have control over; they're already fixed into place.

This means that our destination is a place that already exists and the way to get there has already been mapped out with precision.

already exists and the way to get there has already been mapped out with precision. The only thing needed of us is preparation. It will be very disappointing for us if we get to our destination and find out that we failed to pack our things. What a horrible vacation that would be! Or better yet, what useless expectation in waiting to reach our destiny when upon getting there, we realize we are not equipped. Reaching our destiny alone isn't enough; we must be prepared to handle what destiny has for us.

Preparation—Where is God saying you should go? What passion or drive has He given you? What people has He brought into your life to travel with you—no matter if they're traveling with you the entire way or if you're dropping them off on the way? What lessons have you learned?

Passion—What, when thinking about it, causes you to become righteously angry or empathetic when you see or hear *others* going through it? When these feelings arise, you can't figure out why. You may ask yourself, "Why am I so concerned about this?"

Purpose—Your righteous anger and empathetic feelings will cause you to move toward your purpose. Crunching out this information is your GPS (generalized purpose search). It may not be accurate to the point, but it will give you a generalized area. Passion will help you navigate to your destination.

Keys to safe traveling:

- Plan ahead. Seek out your destination. (What problem am I here to solve?)
- Remember your reason for going (to help others). Don't get caught up in the scenery (trials of life).
- Stick to the road (passion). Do not overthink or turn from it. Your destination has been God-quested.

- Don't pull over on dark roads (unwise counsel); go somewhere well lit (wise counsel).
- Don't drive on an empty tank (fill up on education, learning, wisdom).
- Oh yeah, and most important, do not pick up strangers or hitchhikers (those who are not meant to go and cannot go with you to your destination. They will only slow you down. They see success and purpose and want to jump on the bandwagon).

Station 8—
Preparation for Success

"Preparation is pre-pairing the most congruent and best assembled elements that will lead to a successful whole and finished product."

I love the story of the two farmers who prayed for rain. Both needed a good downpour because the land was dry. They prayed the same prayer, and God sent rain. However, one farmer, after praying, went out and prepared his field. The other farmer did not. Who do you think benefited from the initial prayer and the answer? The farmer who prepared, of course. This story isn't much different from what happens in our lives.

We hope and pray for things to come, but how many people prepare for their arrival? A husband and wife, when expecting a newborn baby, will usually prepare their home for the infant. They set up the infant's room, paint the walls, and assemble the nursery bed, among other things. Once that child begins to crawl and walk, they take extra measures and precautions to administer further safety and protection. What could happen if those same parents were negligent in preparing their home?

The child may be injured or worse. Preparation is a key ingredient in succeeding in any meaningful endeavor.

Steps to Preparation

Preparation for success is integral to producing fruit from the seeds we plant. What are some steps to preparing for success? We can come to this conclusion by observing the nature and habits of a farmer. The first step to her preparation is conceiving of a vision, an idea of what she desires to plant and harvest. Likewise, we need an idea to plant that will eventually produce a harvest.

I can speak for myself in that I had an idea to write a book to help people reform and renew their minds. It starts with an idea or a thought. What are you expecting? Envision it, see it, and know it. Walk it out, measure it, test it—do whatever helps you build on the idea. The farmer wakes up early and gets started early. She isn't hesitant or slothful. All farmers know they have an allotted amount of time to have a vision, prepare the vision, plant the vision, and harvest the vision. Time is of the essence.

The next step after an idea or vision is to plow the soil. Being sure that the soil is able to provide the best sustenance for the seeds is essential to the farmer's success. Hard ground is not the best supporting material or environment for the seeds' growth. Plowing the ground is a process of pulling dirt from the bottom and bringing it to the top. This allows more nutrients to settle at the surface.

Similar to this is the mind and heart. As the Bible illustrates, seeds in the soil of our hearts can come in four different forms. The first form is seed falling by the wayside. Seeds falling by the wayside are ideas which aren't given the chance to take root. This is like an idea that is dismissed immediately without further thought. The second form is seed landing on rocky ground.

In this case, it takes root, but there isn't enough earth to sustain it. This translates into an idea that is accepted but abandoned because of negativity and difficulty. The idea fails because the roots are too shallow. Third, seeds that are planted are choked out by weeds. This is an idea that is choked out by fear, doubt, and pressure. Finally, there is the seed that falls on fertile ground and grows roots long enough to support it until maturation.

Sometimes in our lives, there are things residing at the bottom of our hearts that can help us if brought to the surface. It will take work to bring things to the surface, but the idea is to try. A current issue can be solved if we can remember an older issue of similar concern and how we dealt with that. Most great ideas come from something lying at the bottom of a person's heart. If we think about the ideas that have changed our world, we can see that they came at a time when the need for advancement was at its greatest.

Bad situations have a tendency to bring things to the surface. This process of bringing nutrients to the surface is called plowing, as mentioned previously. Plowing is breaking the top layer of the soil and going deeper where the best soil resides. After the soil has been plowed and the nutrients pulled to the surface, a harrow is used to break up the clods of dirt, smooth out the soil to a flat surface, and disengage roots. Pulling things to the surface of the heart will oftentimes bring up memories or thoughts that are unfruitful to the task at hand.

For instance, if we have an idea and think back on our experiences, sometimes we can bring up a moment of failure from which we learned how to persevere and triumph, but the root of fear may still be attached to that good soil or memory. Therefore, that root has to be disengaged if we want to receive the full benefit of the soil or thought that has been plowed. Also, this process flattens out what should be our focus and helps in moving out what is of little help. Not everything that we've been through will help in every situation, so it's important to recognize what helps and what doesn't help.

Furrows are the neatly created rows that look like long, small mounds. While we remove the unwanted things from the soil of our hearts, we are simultaneously placing into order and pinpointing exactly what we will need to have a successful harvest. The rows keep the plants off of the ground, giving the roots room to grow and helping prevent the plant from drowning. When sustenance to support an idea is brought to the surface or from outside sources, those thoughts supporting the idea must be placed and orchestrated in order. There is nothing worse than having a great idea and no structured plan to implement it.

Components to an idea must be placed in order. Making a plan pulls the idea off the ground and prevents it from dragging along. Sometimes, an idea can drown under the weight of too much information, which can make the idea seem no longer feasible, much like entry barriers and bureaucratic paperwork. After harrowing, the seed can then be planted. The seed is obviously the idea. Planting an idea between the lines of a plan will almost always see it germinate into fruitfulness.

With a seed that is planted, it's not wise to continuously obstruct its growth by constantly removing and replanting it. Likewise, once an idea is planted in a plan; it's not wise to continue to totally reconstruct the plan. It's best to clean up the plan when it's needed—as the farmer would clean up her rows—but to never take the seed out of the groundwork of the original plan. There will be weeds that'll grow in our fields, which we must remove. Plans and especially our hearts aren't always weed-proof.

That is why cultivating is extremely important in farming. Cultivating machinery is used for weeding the field without disturbing the crops. There will be weeds that will try to gain control over our fields, but we must be diligent in eradicating them. After the seed is planted, the next step is to make sure that it's getting enough water and sunlight. Sunlight is equivalent to inspiration, and water is equivalent to knowledge.

We need to continuously pour inspiration and motivation, as well as knowledge, on our ideas each day. Knowledge is the information about how to implement the idea. Finally, we have the threshing. Threshing is when grain is separated from the stalk. It's a way of acquiring the edible inner parts by beating the worthless outer.

It is done on a floor called a threshing floor, which is either hard dirt or boards fit tightly together so that the grain cannot pass through. The place of threshing the grain is located close to the door of the barn so that the worthless chaff, which is lighter, will blow away; the good grain will stay inside, because it is heavier. This beating or threshing process draws similarities with our idea or plan in that we can't hope to produce the best final product in a plan without a little scrutinizing, critical thinking, and hardship. If we skip this step, the idea or plan may not be as good as it could've been if there had been a beating process, which separates the worthless details from the details that stick. Many great entertainers and artists may have creative ideas, but to make these ideas the best they can possibly be, they scrutinize and examine the details until they come down to the best product.

The key is to be flexible. We must refrain from becoming too attached to the original idea. The first and original idea is always a starting point, but it isn't the final product. It's a place to begin and build upon, but it isn't a place to end. This means that the idea should be kept close to the door of the heart, so that it's easier to change what needs to be changed. Most authors have trouble letting an original idea go when writing something they personally enjoy.

After editing and scrutinizing their work, they realize that some changes need to be made. Allowing the work to enter the deep parts of the heart may prove to be difficult later on if there is a need to tweak and change a few things. Hence, it's good to keep in mind the need for flexibility. If this is done diligently, you will eventually acquire the best fruit from your labor. There is, however, a disclaimer.

One summer, I helped my mentor plant a vegetable and fruit garden. What I discovered was that although every plant was planted in the same soil at the same time and received the same sunlight and the same amount of water, not every plant made it to maturation. The point is this: just because you follow these steps does not mean that every idea will succeed. Some will, and some will not, but if you plant enough ideas, one is bound to take root and grow.

Preparing or Pre-Pairing

To prepare means to pair together the best possible combinations beforehand to reach the desired outcome. In childhood, we're generally taught how to pair together integrity, hard work, perseverance, respect, and responsibility. These qualities are ingredients for success later on in life. However, some people either miss out on being taught these principles or fail to implement them. One thing is for sure, and that is these people are usually unsuccessful. To be successful, we need to search out the best ingredients and piece together those qualities.

The finest business consists of the best ingredients assembled beforehand. This is why I like to assemble puzzles. Putting together puzzles is one of my hobbies. I understand that the course of putting together a puzzle will be tedious if I don't prepare first. I prepare by picking out the edge pieces and then assembling them.

Afterward, I choose a section of the picture and decide which pieces best resemble the color, shade, texture, shape, and intrinsic qualities that will give away a clue. This is my preparation; I pre-pair the pieces that I believe will work. We must approach our life and dreams in the same way. We want to pair together the best possibilities to see the best results possible.

Preparing Friendships and Associations

Sometimes, success is even contingent upon piecing together the best group of friends and associates. This is preparing for success. We are who we hang around. I see it all too often; people want to befriend individuals based on their reputation and not their character. This is a big mistake that most, if not all, successful people fail to make.

> If you feel like you don't fit in, maybe it's because your destiny is too large to try to fit it in small places like between the opinions and subjective thoughts of others.

I believe that everyone can learn from this. We must prepare for our future, not to get others to like us or be accepted into the in crowd. Sometimes, the eagerness to belong or fit in will get in the way of our preparation for success. The desire to fit in isn't the best attitude to carry around. If you feel like you don't fit in, maybe it's because your destiny is too large to try to fit it in small places like between the opinions and subjective thoughts of others. Opinions and subjective thoughts equate to what we know as reputation.

Reputation is strictly what others think about us. In high school, we all wanted a good and positive reputation, which translated to what others thought of us; it was all about popularity. We wanted to be around the people everyone knew or be the person everyone knew. The focus was on the person speaking and not on what the person was saying. Sad to say, this mentality hasn't subsided for some of us. Successful people don't flock toward mere reputation based on public demand and liking. They give their attention to anyone who is speaking with substance. The wise lend their ear to anyone and everyone, knowing that they can learn from all. They don't surround themselves with reputation but with character.

As I said earlier, if you feel like you don't fit in, you are probably trying to squeeze between the opinions and subjective thoughts of others. I dealt with this myself until I found out that where I wanted to be accepted wasn't large enough to contain my destiny. This isn't to sound arrogant or prideful, but it's the truth, and I know others can relate. Now I'm in the place I need to be and working on filling up some space in this great sea of awesome people by increasing my knowledge, wisdom, and understanding.

All of this is said both to encourage and to show that the disposition of wanting to belong to a certain group isn't always the best for your given situation. God will begin to prepare you for your destiny at an early age. As I look back on my adolescent life, I recognize all of the struggles and pains that I've gone through as building blocks for where I am now. All of the things that I go through now are building blocks for me to succeed at a later date. Everything in life is about preparation.

Childhood Preparation

My parents taught me to take care of my possessions. It started with toys and clothing and has transitioned into other things that I possess. I can remember as I was growing up seeing toys that children's parents would give them lying out in the yard. Children would receive so many gifts in December, but by March, most of the pieces were either broken or misplaced. How children's characters are prepared is important to their future; their character will determine the kind of life they will have.

At this transition of my life, most of the people I grew up with and went to school with are in the process of defining themselves for the rest of their lives. As I look at those individuals and remember how they behaved as children, I am astonished that most of them primarily behave the same way, but only to another dynamic. The kids who made excuses when they were young make excuses when they're old. The kids who had low self-esteem when they were younger still exhibit a form of low self-esteem now that they're older.

I've seen children whose parents gave them everything that they wanted when they were younger, and as adults, they still believe they are supposed to get any and everything they want. People seldom grow out of the characters they exhibited as children. If a kid is mischievous, he or she will probably be mischievous as an adult. There are a few people who will recognize their character as unsavory and will change it on their own, but this is very rare. People will generally stick with the attitude, disposition, and character they were raised with and prepared to operate in as an adult.

My parents weren't strict, but I respected them. I spent many lonely days in my backyard with a basketball in my hand. As I was growing up, my house was the hub for sports, because I had a bigger backyard than the kids with whom I played. I also had a basketball goal. Those days were fun, playing games from sunup to sundown. However, when the fun wasn't at my house, it was at my friend's house down the street, and this was where things got a little difficult.

I would have to ask my parents if I could go play with my friends. If they said yeah, I went, but sometimes, my friends wanted to move to another location. I had to go back home and ask my parents again if I could go to the new location. This was quite embarrassing, being that none of the other guys had to do this. Sometimes, once I got back to where I had last left my friends, everyone would be gone.

That was tough on a young boy who only wanted to be with the guys, but I learned accountability from it. I learned integrity and honesty, because I could have left without my parents' consent, but the idea of letting my parents down was worse than feeling embarrassed. I always believed that if my parents were going to have faith in me, I couldn't disappoint them. Now in my adult years, I see that accountability and keeping my word is extremely important, especially in this day where contracts are prevalent because people lack accountability and integrity. Trying to fit in and be a part of the in crowd would've left me without the valuable lessons that I have today.

One of the reasons that our world is suffering is because people lack good and basic character qualities. It may be because many people would like to fit in and belong, but as you can see, fitting in, belonging, or being accepted leaves many people with less than what they could've gained. I'm not saying that the sense of wanting to belong is a bad thing. God built in us the ability, need, and desire to be

> Establishing basic character qualities is one important step to preparation for a successful life, which then leads to contribution to the world.

social, but that sense of belonging cannot interfere with us being at our best. Establishing basic character qualities is one important step to preparation for a successful life, which then leads to contribution to the world.

Succeeding in smaller things adds up to succeeding in more significant things. Did you suffer from timidity as a child? You were probably preparing for timidity as an adult. Were you selfish as a child? You are probably going to be selfish in your adult years. Were you overcome with jealousy as a child? You're possibly jealous now as an adult. Were you caring, giving, responsible, respectful, or honest as a child? You are more than likely the same way as an adult. Either way, preparation in anything starts early in the course of life or the life of your given aim of success.

Preparing for Change

Let's transition our focus to our current state. We can't change the hands of time, but we can change the damage that has been done. It's just like working on an old vintage vehicle; there are some parts that need to be replaced, because some of the parts are going to be defective. The use of them probably seemed logical at one point, but over time, they have proven to be more of a nuisance than anything else. They just don't work like they used to.

We can use the example of the pity party. The pity party that someone once threw as a cute five-year-old has since turned him or her into an annoying, crybaby adult, who knows how to ruin the mood if not given what he or she wants. This part may have worked a while ago, but since then, it has become a nuisance because the pity party doesn't quite work like it used to. This part is defective and needs to be replaced. This adult needs to learn the proper way of communicating needs and wants.

Some defective parts are obvious, and others need some searching out to be revealed, but we all have defective parts that need replacing. Some parts that used to work could use some upgrading. For a long time, I disliked to loan out my belongings to anyone who would ask to borrow them. I knew they wouldn't take care of my belongings as well as I took care of them; nevertheless, it's praiseworthy to loan our possessions to help meet the needs of others. I slowly but surely developed this mind-set, and truthfully, I feel more liberated now, but I have to admit, as I suspected, not everyone cherished my belongings as much as I did.

This isn't to harp on, because this is nothing more than a defective part. They have some character issues to change within them also, but I needed people like this in my life because I developed greater patience, as well as a greater expression of grace. All of this has helped make me into and prepare me to be the person that I am today. It all begins with preparing for and wanting change. The parts that I needed to change were my attitude, lack of trust in people, and, in some ways, selfishness.

I had to identify this mind-set and put the pieces together to see the greater picture. This greater picture identified my errors and areas in need of correction. Oftentimes, once the pieces are placed together, the greater picture helps us understand more clearly the need for change. It also helps bring the foresight that this particular change can and will result in a sense of greater responsibility to ourselves, to our families, and to the world.

Women of Chastity

When opportunity comes knocking, we don't want to be caught off guard. We may not know exactly when it'll come, but it will come. Our only duty is to be ready. This reminds me of the story of the ten women of chastity. Five were wise, and five were foolish. All ten women went out during the night to wait on an arrival; five of them were wise and brought extra oil to fuel their lamps. The other five were foolish and didn't bring extra oil for their lamps.

The ten women waited as the arrival tarried. They slumbered and slept in eager waiting, but the wise women were ready for what happened next. At once, the expected arrived, and the women readied themselves to go out and accost the arrival. As they rose from their sleep, the wise women grabbed their still-burning lamps and began to walk. They were interrupted by the foolish women who didn't bring extra oil, as their lamps had burned out.

They asked the wise women for oil, but the wise women refused their pleas. They convinced the foolish women to go and buy their own oil. The foolish women left, and when they came back, they were amazed to find that the wise women and the expected arrival had come and gone. This story is an illustration that shows that being prepared is essential to life.[5]

Don't Fool Yourself ... Prepare!

I learned a valuable lesson while in college, and the lesson was, prepare even when you think you have it. Being the president of the

FCA (Fellowship of Christian Athletes) required me to speak before my teammates, coaches, and visitors. I can remember the first time I took the stand as the president. I went in confident that I would know what to say. I came out not so sure.

Being the quasi-perfectionist that I am, I was a bit embarrassed at my performance. I had the mind-set that if I spoke, I wanted to be heard and make a difference, but it's hard to make a difference if your words come out in stutters, slips, and incomplete thoughts. I should've learned my lesson, but that wasn't the last time that happened because of my lack of preparation. I continued to fool myself, saying, "Okay, I know the routine now; I know what to say." Can I get a big, "Yeah, right!"? I still blew it after thinking that I understood the flow. Those thoughts still haunt me to this day. The lesson that I learned was never to underestimate the value of preparation—even in the thing in which we believe we will succeed. Don't fool yourself. Be smart; be prepared.

Action Steps

1. Conceive of an idea, vision, goal, or dream.
2. Determine the soil of your heart. Do you know that you can accomplish this idea, vision, goal, or dream? If not, stop now and recondition your beliefs.
3. Ponder and muse over what you've accomplished—your successes and triumphs, small or large. This will help in conditioning your heart for planting. Read biographies of your heroes, and see what they persevered through to reach their level of success. Many of them began with nothing.
4. Disengage fear or any bad thoughts from your triumphal experiences.
5. Construct a thorough plan, and make your goals feasible.
6. Once the plan is set, leave it, tweak it only if you have to.
7. Don't wait for opportunity; prepare for it to come.

Station 9—
Determination and Persistence

"Determination and persistence support one another and keep
each other from falling."

Whenever I hear the word *determination*, I hear the words *deter* and *terminate*. Determination is a strong word, invoking images of an android walking around with a big gun on its hip. *Webster's New Explorer Dictionary* says *deter* means "to discourage and prevent from acting"[6] and of course, *terminate* means "to bring or come to an end."[7] So in determination, we have an action that brings an end to any thought or deed that is causing discouragement. In the same word, there is the word *determine*.

To determine is to decide something or to settle something conclusively. In determination, the first step is to decide that what you want to get done will get done and that nothing is going to hold you back from accomplishing it. So what we have is a decision that is made that will bring an end to any and everything that is blocking your passage to reaching your goal. The true definition of determination, however, is firmness of purpose or fixed purpose. People who have claimed personal success will always have a fixed thought of what they want their life to be like and what results they would like to see. This is a staple of success.

Make a Decision

Finding the resolve to continue regardless of barriers and stumbling blocks is the essence of determination. As you can see, I find joy looking into words to gain greater clarity, and one word that stands out in comprehending the trait of determination is the word *resolve*. To resolve means to make a decision. This is simply what determination is, making a decision. Harriet Tubman resolved that she would escape and help others escape the brutal reality of slavery.

Deciding that she would help slaves flee to safety and daring never to turn back developed into determination. Bill Gates determined that every home would have a personal computer, and we see what became of that. Henry Ford determined that the old horse-propelled carriages would be replaced with engine-propelled cars. Bruce Lee determined that anyone who wanted to learn martial arts should be taught. By all these people, standards were drawn that still stand to this day because they were determined. They had a resolve and never let that decision go or dissipate.

Persistence

What fits nicely alongside determination is persistence. Sometimes, these two words can be thought to mean the same thing, but they are different in meaning. Determination, of course, is a firmness of purpose, but persistence is continuing steadily despite problems or difficulties. So determination sets a resolve, but persistence is what sees the resolve through to completion. So, for example, if I am a marathon runner, I would need both determination and persistence.

Determination would play a role in helping me make the decision to run 26.2 miles and that nothing is going to stop me once I take to the course. Persistence plays its part when I become fatigued and my body begins to ache. Persistence is strongly persuading myself not to quit but to push through to the end. Determination is as important as persistence. One isn't more significant than the other, because we need determination to start the process and persistence to finish the process.

Persistence can be seen in this illustration. You may have seen grass blades that find and push their way through the cracks of a concrete sidewalk. We know that the grass wasn't there at first, so how did it get there? Or better yet, how did it push through the concrete?

Well, most definitely, the grass made its way through to see the light of day by persistence. The world is like concrete, which to the grass was an oppressor. In all forms of oppression, there is always a way out, and there is, over time, somewhere where we can find a break in the oppression of the world and fight through just like the blades of grass. Oppression never lasts forever. Although it is consistent throughout the world, your personal life will

> In all forms of oppression, there is always a way out, and there is, over time, somewhere where we can find a break in the oppression of the world and fight through just like the blades of grass.

see a break, a crack, where the daylight can be seen, and it is your duty to fight and push through.

It's your duty to take advantage of the present opportunity to break through. Life is a fight. A war is strategic, but victory usually lies in persistence. We must push until there is a breakthrough or manifestation as the result of our persistence. Ironically, it was pushing that birthed us.

Our mothers pushed until we were birthed and gave us the ability to have uninhibited life. Our dreams, goals, and visions are the same way; we must push our goals through and give them uninhibited life. Of course, it will be painful, just ask any mom, but the pain is worth it once you see the dream that you first conceived of and then pushed to birth.

Persistence and Tug-of-War

I imagine persistence as a lonely game of tug-of-war with the world, which is your opponent. You're on one side, and the world is on the other. Who is on the world's side? The naysayers, those who envy, fear, worry, social disadvantages, indecision, and so on. The rope that you're holding in your hands is your dream.

There's always going to be a tug-of-war with the world over your dreams, because the world will do its best to defeat you. Usually, it seems as if everyone is either encouraging your opponent or is on your opponent's side. Sometimes, striving for victory and achieving your dream can be a lonely game. The world pulls and pulls, trying to snatch your dream away. What happens with some people is that once the world gives a good heave on the rope, they feel the tug, and when they begin to fall forward, they let go.

Out of fear of falling, failing, hurting themselves, or being embarrassed, they let go; this is what the world wants. Now the world has your dream, and the world has won. Those people who achieve and reach their dreams are the ones who felt the tug by the world and sensed the inevitability of falling down but didn't mind if they did. They didn't mind if they failed or hurt themselves or even embarrassed themselves.

> Those people who achieve and reach their dreams are the ones who felt the tug by the world and sensed the inevitability of falling down but didn't mind if they did.

All they knew was that they were going to get up off of the ground with their rope still in their hands.

They were not going to let their dreams go, and as they emerged from the ground dirty, bloodied, and even embarrassed, they were still in the game. See, the rules of the game of holding on to your dream are a little different than those of the normal game of tug-of-war. In the normal rules, the first person or team to cross the middle of the halfway point loses, but in this real-life case, it's the first person who relinquishes their power. Thankfully, sometimes in life, once the spectators have seen how tenacious we are in reaching our dream and how we have fallen but yet will not let go of the dream, they come along and assist us. Now we aren't alone in the struggle; we have others who have gone through the same game and won their own individual battles, those who realize the difficulty of our current situation.

People usually are not going to help if they don't see that we are dedicated and persistent in reaching our dream. My mentor once said to me, "Everyone isn't going to be as excited about your dream as you are." What I also received from that was that people may not be as excited about our dream, but the idea is to never give up because once they see the dream unfolding, they will want to help. Naturally, people desire to be around success or be a part of a success story. Never let go of your dream. Hold on for dear life. Help will come. Be persistent.

The Strength to Hold On

In tug-of-war, you need strong legs, strong arms, and a really strong back. You need strong legs to hold your position and push back and away from the negativity that the world can bring. Holding your position in life will become important when others come and try to convince you that what you're aspiring to do is impossible. You need strong legs to take a stand against the negativity and naysayers. Sometimes in life, you need to take a stand in the hopes of showing the world that it will no longer push you around and snatch away your dreams.

Charles T. Robinson Jr.

Resolve to take a stand. The only way to strengthen your legs is to engage them in exercise. Exercise your right to stand in the freedom and liberty of reaching your dream or goal. In the same right, you need strong arms to hold the load of the demands that life

> It's important to never allow someone else to form your world for you, because oftentimes, they will construct something that will constrict you.

brings. Life can become heavy, and strong arms are a must if you hope to hold your weight and press the world away from you.

We will not accept the thoughts and attitudes of the world because the world's attitudes and thoughts will fail us every time. We also need strong arms to keep a good grasp on our dreams. It's important to never allow someone else to form your world for you, because oftentimes, they will construct something that will constrict you. Form your own world, and don't allow anyone else to form it for you. Generally, people are not going to want more for you than they want for themselves.

This is sad to say, but it's true. I see it every day. The only time you'll find someone pushing you along to fulfill your dreams is if they're secure in their achievements or if they want to see you succeed out of the love they have for you. People who don't care much about you won't want you to have more than they have. They definitely aren't going to help you produce more than they can produce or succeed beyond the limits that they have set for themselves. Therefore, take the pleasure in forming your own world.

The good thing about this is if the world you form is too small or too complex, it'll be your fault and no one else's. You can place the blame on yourself. Too often, we allow the opinions and thoughts of others to shape our world. We are supposed to care about our neighbors but not so much about what they think about us. Everyone has an opinion about something, so don't be distraught when someone offers you their negative presumptions.

How do we deal with the cynicism of others? We continue the development of our arms so that we may pull ourselves above the cynicism. Finally, we build a strong back, which is very important. Our back muscles play an important role in the pulling motion.

To pull back our dream from the world, we must have a backbone. Once again, we must not become frail under the circumstances and cower away. This is exactly what the world wants; it wants us to become cowards. I know *coward* is a strong word, but I want to evoke a strong reaction, because when we allow our dreams to be taken

> To pull back our dream from the world, we must have a backbone.

away, this is exactly what we become, cowards. We must be tenacious in pursuing our dreams and be their sole protector.

Our dreams should be like a newborn infant needing our protection and guidance at every step. We wouldn't leave an infant to fend and care for itself, would we? No, we wouldn't. So then why would we allow our dreams to go unprotected? We wouldn't allow everyone to hold our newborn baby, but we allow people to hold the fate of our dreams in their mouths, bringing up every bad situation that could possibly happen or why our dreams shouldn't happen. We don't want people speaking badly of our dreams and giving discouraging advice.

It's important to nurse and protect the dream by watching who we allow to be around it. Don't be careless; you can't tell everyone about your dream. Some people may seem genuine but are secretly harboring strong feelings of envy and jealousy toward you. We must clothe the dream with new ideas and concepts, feed the dream by acquiring more knowledge on the particular subject, and burp and clean the dream by removing the things that won't work, but most important, we must interact with our dream so that it can evolve and grow.

Technique to Winning the Game

The game of tug-of-war is based on strength, tenacity, and technique. We put our heels into the ground, lean back, and pull hand over fist, all the while being careful not to relinquish any rope that we have gained. I cannot emphasize this enough. Refrain from succumbing to the demands of the world when it comes to your dreams. Continue to pull and gain more territory and confidence.

The more rope you hold, the less your opponent has to work with; therefore, gain as much confidence as you can. It will support you fulfilling your dream, and the world will not have enough grip on your dream to snatch it away. This is important to get, because each year, there are many people who give up on their dreams because of all the things mentioned above. Do not become a part of the statistics. Every year, publications say how many businesses fail to succeed past five years, and some people become afraid to start their own business out of fear of failure.

I must've been extremely optimistic or extremely gullible, because I always managed to think that those statistics wouldn't apply to me. I've been optimistic about a few things in my life. As a young black male, I was technically entailed to be an at-risk youth. An at-risk youth is a child who has or may have problems with his or her development that may affect later learning. Granted, I did fail the first grade, but that didn't shape my outcome.

After repeating the first grade, I never looked back. I grew up in a decent neighborhood, but drugs were all around me. I could've gotten caught up in that lifestyle, but I didn't, which is a testament to the loving, saving grace of Jesus Christ and a testament to my parents' rearing of me. The at-risk characteristics passed me. However true it may have been, I never saw myself that way.

I was quite astonished when someone told me that I possibly could have been labeled at-risk, simply because I never saw myself in that light. Self-image is crucial to success, and because I saw myself as determined not to end up like the people I saw in my neighborhood and was persistent in becoming successful, I am here today writing a book on building minds so that we can individually help build others. I applied the technique and didn't let my dream go. I held on for dear life despite the bumps, bruises, and embarrassments.

The Time Is Now

We have heard the person who has made the claim of what they are determined to do one day. Someone may say, "I am determined to learn how to play the piano one day." That's awesome that this person has the fixed thought of wanting to play the piano, but that fixed thought is going to be just that, fixed. Thoughts are not going anywhere until we actually put our hands to the plow. Thought without action is worthless.

Faith is a fixed thought, and another term for determination. When we have faith, we have a constant, unwavering belief that something will happen. For those who have trouble having a fixed mind will rarely receive what they think they want. We don't want to get caught up in the one-day mind-set. That's another term for procrastination. The best time is always now. Refrain from putting things off that could be taken care of at the present moment, and remember, first determine, and then act.

Determination and Imagination

Determination is closely linked with imagination. If we can see our dream by imagining it with specific detail, we will have greater determination to strive after that thing. We see what lies ahead of us. Exercise your imagination by fixing in your mind the final outcome of your dream or goal. When you do this, the mind will strive to manifest physically what it sees spiritually.

Remember, the greatest desire of those things unseen is the ability to be seen and express themselves. This is a sure way to motivate yourself and increase your determination. Determination will cross over to work ethic. The more determined we are, the harder we'll work. Work is the necessary evil of drawing what has been imagined out of the dark abyss and into the light.

Once we think about something intensively and believe that we can have it in faith, it is created in the spiritual realm, just like that! Our only job is then to keep it there by continuing to focus and work on drawing it out of the darkness. We must have a willingness to draw it out of the darkness and a keen sense of zeal, passion, and urgency in seeing it to maturation. Over time and by hard work, it will appear.

> Work is the necessary evil of drawing what has been imagined out of the dark abyss and into the light.

Everything starts with a thought or idea, and in this case, the word for that is, *determine*. Determine what you will create in the darkness of the unseen.

Determine what you will draw out of the abyss by hard work. Determine what you will keep in mind and make manifest. Hard work and persistence go hand in hand because we should be determined to work diligently toward excellence. Excellence isn't easy to come by and takes a lot of work to produce, but this is persistence at its best. It means never settling for less but always striving to do the best job possible. This should be our attitude in anything that we do. We should develop the mind-set of excellence because this particular mind-set doesn't come overnight. This mind-set is something that needs work, and the only way to get there is through persistence.

Excellence in Persistence

On any sports team, the idea is for everyone to be in the same state of mind. Everyone should have the same determination, the same fixed mind-set. That mind-set is governed toward teamwork and winning. This is ideal. Usually, however, there will only be a few players on the team who would qualify as persistent. These are the players who stay after practice to work on their weak points. They have the concept of team and determination, but they have taken it a step further and have also brought in persistence to be the best player that they can possibly be. Persistence works in every area of our lives. The best athletes, performers, and artists didn't get that way by chance or luck. They got that way through sheer persistence, by tweaking and refining their craft.

Success Is a Process

I've made this statement before and I'll make it again: there really are no secrets to success. Many people would like to think so, but it's simply not true. All people who have reached success have gotten there by determination and persistence. This generation is far past the microwave generation in regard to how ridiculously fast we like to receive gratification. Those individuals who understand that success doesn't come from instant gratification but from longsuffering and persistence with a mind of resolve are the ones who reach true success.

People who try to get meaningful things quickly usually lose them at the same rate, because it takes a certain mind-set to gain meaningful things legitimately, and that mind-set qualifies that person to keep what he or she has gained. For the person who gained success frivolously will only lose it because he or she does not understand the laws governing success. He who is a good steward over a little will be qualified to be a steward over much. As for he who is a poor steward over little, why should he be trusted over bigger and greater things? If anything, as it has been said, success is a mystery because no one really knows why the principles of success work as they do. It's only wise to follow the principles.

Before people were able to understand the complexities of gravity, no one would bet against its power; they respected the power. The same is true for determination and persistence and for all the success principles. Success is a mystery that doesn't hide from anyone but the unknowledgeable. So, as a joke, I guess I can say I hope you enjoy and appreciate a good mystery novel, because that is simply what success is: a mystery.

The Road of Persistence

Failure is the town we drop by while navigating the road of persistence. Failures are a must. We fail not because we want to but because we have to. Even if we really are determined, our persistence may sometimes wane on us, so we need to stop by the nearest town to refuel. God knows the exact moment to bring failure into our lives. It will give us the opportunity to check under the hood, clean off the windshield, and refuel.

We should check under the hood to see if our plan needs a tune-up. We may need to adopt a different outlook. Maybe what we see isn't something that is going to be totally different from our original plan, but we may need to tweak something or add something in the same fashion we would add oil to an engine. Sometimes, we may need to clean the windshield because our view has becoming blurry, meaning we need to regain focus. Lastly, the fuel gauge may be creeping over to empty, so we need to fuel up on persistence.

Sometimes, we may become a little complacent, and there is nothing like failure to bring us back to reality. Failure is always the best tool to ground the person who has the big head. Failure brings everything back into perspective; we are able to see more clearly once our head is out of the clouds. In the beginning, the road of persistence can be quite bumpy, but as we travel this road, it becomes a much smoother ride and more enjoyable. Eventually in life, we will begin to appreciate the pit stops at the towns called failure, because we will have the unquestioned chance to be prudent and recheck our route before proceeding.

Going in the Wrong Direction

When we think about being persistent, we usually think that it's a good thing. Persistence can be both good and bad. We've discussed some of the good, so let's take a look at the bad. Persistence can be bad because over time, we can unconsciously develop bad habits by way of persistence. If we're always running late, this may develop into persistence in going in the wrong direction. All it takes is a few times to develop this habit, and it becomes a part of our character. This effect can continue to happen long after the initial cause has ceased. We want persistence to work for us and not against us, so go in the correct direction and use the driving force of persistence to propel you forward and not backward.

Action Steps

1. Decide what you want to do, and allow that fire of desire to burn brightly. The greater the desire, the greater and more fixed the determination will become.

2. Don't worry if you can't conjure up much desire for the thing you want to do. This is God's way of communicating with you that this isn't what you are supposed to be doing. So find your true passion.

3. The biggest part is to make a firm decision and stick to it, so make the decision and don't look back.

4. Push through any negativity that may come your way. Resist

it with all your might, and strive to the completion of your goal.

5. Discredit any naysayers by doing what they said couldn't be done.

6. Take this time to ask yourself a few questions and add your questions to this list, because you are the best person to question yourself.

7. What are you determined to do?

8. What will you fix your mind to do?

9. What is your level of persistence?

10. Will you give it all that you have?

11. Will you block out all negativity?

Station 10—
Progress

"The road that you're on isn't important. What's important is the direction you're traveling while on the road."

Progress is a steady process, and you have to love it. Progress starts small; therefore, we should not forsake our humble beginnings. People make promises claiming that whatever we want can easily be obtained if we do a few things to bring it about. Those promises are empty and leave the unsuspected victim with a short stick. Nature proves the fast success principles to be futile.

Nature takes its time, and over time, it produces seed after its own kind. We will never see a harvest grow overnight; therefore, whatever seeds we plant into our lives will grow, but only over time. The seeds that we plant, whether of diligence or carelessness, will produce after their own kind. This is progress whether good or bad. There is a special consideration of time for everything, so time is a prerequisite.

This is why we should redeem the time in this day, because this day is full of vices that are stealing our time. This wasted time could be used to improve ourselves, our families, and our communities, which includes our world. God has given us the special ability to redeem our time, by giving us the ability to think. If we can think, we can devise a plan to improve our situation. God has specifically graced the human race with this awesome gift. And it's the only thing that separates humans from the rest of God's creations.

If we forfeit our ability to think, that sets us on the level of God's lower creations. In this case, the person may have the image of a human but lack the mind that makes one human. So before learning how to redeem the time and progress, we must first learn how to redeem our minds. Nevertheless, progress is a steady process, and what we do with it determines our future.

Progression of Time

Time will progress whether we like it or not. It's constantly rolling and will not stop for anyone. The question then becomes if time steadily progresses, will we progress with it? Time for time's sake will always have positive development. There are no glitches, no hesitations, and no time-outs; there is nothing of the sort, only a steady and gradual revolution of time.

I like to use the analogy of the father and his daughter. A good father will be protective of his daughter, especially from guys who are lurking around possibly wanting to court her. Progress is the offspring of time. They're like father and daughter, so then we must learn to interact with them both. Time is the father, so we must go through the father before we can see his daughter, progress.

How we interact with time determines how much of progress we are going to see. We aren't going to be a jerk with time and hope to see progress. Eh-eh, it's not going to happen. As the adage goes, most women will choose a husband much like their father. If this is true, progress will observe the characteristics of her father, who is time, and this will determine whether she desires you or not.

In this case, I'm referring to positive and good progress. Father Time is viewed by his daughter as the catalyst to the continuing process of development. If you're looking for progress, but you look nothing like her father—a continuing process of development—she will overlook you. Time is what you make of it, and progress will always look toward time to see if you're worthy. Therefore, make the best impression with time, and you'll gain its approval to see progress.

Regress

Everything has an opposite, and if it's not progress, it's regress. To regress is to return to an earlier state before the commencement of progress or worse. Whatever may be the area of regress, there is undoubtedly less than what was there previously. As an athlete, I constantly found myself wanting to become stronger and gain more muscle so I was always lifting weights. My body type, however, didn't allow for me to gain much weight.

Most people have no problem gaining weight; their problem is losing weight, but I was just the opposite. If they didn't work out, they would gain weight, and if I didn't work out, I would lose weight. After football, I lost my desire to constantly lift weights, and all that I had worked so hard to gain slid right off me, up to eighteen pounds. I know some people are out there saying, "Wow, I wish my body could do that." Well, I'm saying, "Wow, I wish my body wouldn't do that"—or not so easily at least, but the gist is that I regressed from my progress.

The only way for me to keep my progress is to maintain what I have earned. Just like I did, we usually allow what we have gained to deteriorate because of lack of maintenance. If we don't maintain them, in this fallen world, things will naturally regress, so this life is like pushing a boulder uphill. We can either continue to push or we can stop and maintain our position, but if we sit down, the boulder is going back down the hill, and so long to our hard work and progress.

Charles T. Robinson Jr.

Action Is Not without Problems and Progress

Anything we do that requires activity is progress, and this action is derived from a problem. We have a problem that needs to be solved, so we move to action and end in progress. When we encounter a problem that we want to do something about, we take action and begin to move toward a solution, even if that thing that we would like to do is destructive. The action toward doing something destructive, to the person, is still progress. Even destructive actions derive from a problem, though the individual is using the wrong mental faculty to handle the problem.

I have seen a common mistake in which assumptions are made based on messages in the form of text messaging or e-mail. The way we communicate with one another is as much body language and voice tone and pitch as it is words. Sometimes, text doesn't do us any justice in this area, so we often make conclusions based on an assumption of the intent of the sender. The correct mental faculty to use in this situation is to think, *Maybe the person didn't mean it as it's written. Allow me to call them personally and see.* I have experienced this, and luckily, I had the gumption to call that person personally.

Even in this instance, it can be seen that taking action to call my friend because of a problem ended in progress on my part. Action and progress go hand in hand. Therefore, if there is no action, there is no progress. The piano novice will not learn how to play the piano if he or she doesn't take action toward practicing. Whether it's physical practice sitting in front of a real piano or mental practice, mentally going over finger placement and notes, action must be taken.

This can be seen in the most trivial actions. If your arm is trapped underneath your pillow

> Action and progress go hand in hand. Therefore, if there is no action, there is no progress.

140

over a matter of minutes, your arm will go numb. So what do you do? You move it. You had a problem, moved to action, came to a solution, and made progress beginning from the original problem.

Whichever way we choose to view this, the end result is that we need action if we want progress. We encounter problems every day. We live in a problem-filled world. The alarm clock goes off; there's a problem. You may be saying, "Yeah, the problem is that it's buzzing." This is true, but the real problem is that it's time to get up.

So we take the necessary steps to make this happen. Whichever way you may get up—whether you're like a zombie sitting up and stretching forward like Frankenstein making every weird noise that would make crickets seem pleasant or you literally roll out of bed—everyone has their specific action. Another problem arises; where's the breakfast? We take steps to prepare breakfast. Our entire life is full of problems, so I wonder why some of us are so frantic when "real" problems occur.

When solving a problem, we need to find a way to resolve the difficulty or find an answer, which is a solution. One description for a solution is two or more substances mixed together in a fluid. Either description works. When we want to make lemon iced tea, we encounter a problem. The water, tea bags, sugar, ice cubes, and lemon are all separate.

Problems are natural; solutions aren't. So then to solve this problem and make the solution we know as lemon iced tea, we have to combine the elements involved in iced tea. Our arrival at a desirable solution like that of

> Problems are natural; solutions aren't.

iced tea also depends on how we make it. Too much water and it'll be diluted and watery; too much sugar and it'll be too sweet; and too much lemon will make it bitter—the success of the solution depends on how the ingredients are brought together. People who are in financial difficulty can take action and make progress, or they can sit down and do nothing, but the problem will not go away.

Your financial difficulty solution is like the iced tea. You have the creditor, yourself, the telephone, and your personal finances. To make a solution, these ingredients need to come together, but most of the time, people want to keep them separate. That's not how we make progress away from a problem. Also, as with the tea, if people would like to come to a solution, they have to be careful how they make it. Sometimes, conversation in person is better than by telephone. If you're married, maybe your spouse is a better negotiator and more convincing; whatever it may be, the way the ingredients are placed together determines the outcome. Action is not without problems and progress.

Momentum

If you have ever moved from one living arrangement to another, you can understand and appreciate the hassle of packing and unpacking. The writing on the boxes identifies the contents, "Living Room," "Dining Room," "Master Bedroom," "Kitchen," "Kitchen—fragile," and on the box that gets everything thrown in it because you're tired of packing and writing, "Miscellaneous." Once the boxes are in the new house, then the fun begins all over again with unpacking and sorting. I worked for a moving company as a summer job one year, so I've seen it all, packed it all, and unpacked it all. When the guys and I found the best place to park the big rig and threw on our gloves, it was time to go to work.

There was a period of time that signified when we really began to work. In the early process of unloading the trailer, we were trying to warm up, but after about fifteen minutes in, we were rolling; you couldn't stop us. We were making progress, or as some people like to phrase it, we were putting a dent in the (total number of) boxes moved. Sometimes, we would be working so well that we willingly worked into our lunch break. This form of progress shows the law of momentum.

When we have momentum, we have power and are able to develop at an increasing rate. Without any hindrances, the pace will continue to increase. Momentum is excellent in everything we do that is toward reaching success. Success is something that isn't reached easily, so anything that can propel us there is beneficial.

Change

Progress can go down the road of constructive progress or destructive progress. Abraham Lincoln is an example of constructive progress; Adolf Hitler is an example of destructive progress. Both men made progress respectively, but one made constructive progress and the other made destructive progress. If you're on the road of destructive progress (of course not to the extent of a Hitler, but you need change), refrain from proceeding down the road that leads to destruction. People who impede themselves from continuing down the road of destruction can turn back, and the sooner they take this action, the faster they'll come to constructive progress.

The road of destruction is an easy road to follow. Ironically, the easiest roads to walk are those going down a decline, and the hardest roads to walk are those going up on an incline. A destructive path doesn't warrant much effort on our behalf. One bad decision and one second is all it takes to head down this road. A lifetime of bad thinking will get us on this road.

On the other hand, anyone who has traveled the path of success will tell us that this particular path is best to walk if we want to get into shape. Get what into shape? Our minds, that's what. How much strain does a declining path place on our bodies compared to an inclined path? We can get very far on the road of destruction because the natural declining gradient of the road propels our destructive behavior forward. Going up an inclined road, however, we must put effort into walking, and it's not easy. Change is the action that must be taken, and there must be a change in the direction of our thoughts as we educate ourselves.

Motion Alone Isn't Progress

We mustn't get action and motion confused. Action is doing something to reach a purpose; motion is moving from one spot to another. In order to have action, there must be movement, but movement alone will not equate to progress. There must be a distinct goal or purpose in order to have progress. Having a distinct goal puts us into the position of knowing exactly what action to take.

We may have crossed someone who knew they needed change but didn't take the time to pinpoint what kind of change they needed. They didn't want to come to grips with reality. Therefore, they were trying to change by motion and not by action. They were trying to move out of a situation instead of changing themselves for the situation. People who do this are referred to as runners.

They're constantly running from problems, relying on motion and not enough on action. To be clear, motion is trying to change without a distinct plan, moving in whatever direction seems plausible for the time, just to escape the reality of the situation. We've come across people who will blame everyone else, so every time, they come out squeaky clean and self-righteous in all of their ways. They need change. They need to take personal action and cease relying solely on motion to cure their problems.

Steps to Change

Be honest with ourselves. Being self-righteous will only heighten the problem. We have to be honest and know that we need change.

Realize that if we aren't honest with ourselves, in the long run, we aren't hurting anyone but ourselves. We must come to grips with reality concerning this fact.

Take the time for introspection. Search and pinpoint the areas we need change in and write them down. We must diligently search the heart for inconsistencies that aren't agreeable with the person we want to become. We have to be brutally honest.

Confess the problem to a close friend, someone who isn't going to say, "I told you so," or be harsh by saying things like, "Wow, finally!" Even if they're thinking it, they don't need to say it. What they need to do is be supportive. That is the person we need as our accountability.

Go to sleep at night and wake up in the morning knowing that this change will come to fruition. Realizing and learning to cope with the fact that it will be an uphill battle will prepare us for disappointments. Some days will be harder than others, but knowing that we don't have to be perfect is the key. The only thing that matters is that we give consistent and wholesome effort.

Be consistent. Do not miss a day. One day will turn into two and so on. Remember, we're fighting against old habits that we're trying to break; it would behoove us not to give old habits room to grow. We must smother them with consistency and continue to have our mind renewed.

Progressive Setbacks

Progressive setbacks sound like an oxymoron and are exact opposites in meaning and design, but they can work very well together. Our ultimate path in life is never as straight as we would hope. There are some bends, turns, U-turns, and speed bumps that we will stumble upon as we travel. It wouldn't seem wise to say that a setback is a good place to be. Who likes setbacks?

Well, truthfully, the answer to that question is the people who are seasoned and know how a setback is able to boost them forward. These people realize that if they allow a setback to do what it's designed to do

> A setback is an awesome teacher with a degree in where not to go and how not to do it next time.

and be patient, they will come out better than before. A setback is an awesome teacher with a degree in where not to go and how not to do it next time. The setback has thousands of years in training and teaches all those who would like to learn more about reaching higher levels in life. Even those who are content with mediocrity will face setbacks' teachings.

Many have heard about setbacks' classes but are afraid of having to take their course. Some try to avoid this teaching, but in order to graduate to the next level in life, each person needs a certain number of credits earned respective to each individual's needs. It's wise to be an attentive and open student to the teaching of setbacks, because if we're not, we'll see the same course load again. Setbacks teach at all levels in life, from childhood setbacks to the setbacks of a Fortune 500 company, but the trick is to learn and pass with flying colors. What can we do in times of setback?

Well, let's view this question as it would be in a student-teacher relationship. Can you remember when one of your friends had a teacher that you were also destined to have and this particular teacher was on everyone's "F" radar? Can you remember asking your friend questions, and your buddy telling you what to do and what not to do in this teacher's class? Well, I'm your friend.

This is what you want to do in setbacks' class.

1. Listen attentively. Attentive listening in life is opening up our minds to what the setback in our life wants to convey

to us. No setback in life is without a voice. Each situation occurs for a reason, and this reason is so that setback can sit us down and teach.

2. Allow minimum distractions. There are many distractions in life from cell phones to reality television to unnecessary worrying, and each distraction should be kept at bay. Our focus should be so intensely aimed at the teachings of the setback that our attention is diverted by the teaching away from the objects of distraction. Things will tap us on the shoulder and try to amuse us, but we have to remain focused on the task at hand.

3. Pay attention to the teacher only. The teacher is in the front of the classroom, not behind. I say that the teacher is in the front of the classroom and not behind because I am building proximity to where we should be in life and that is in the front row. Once your hands are placed to the plow, don't distract and prohibit yourself by peering back. Many times in life, there are so many voices vying for our attention. Every night, there are hundreds of infomercials that air promising debt-free finances, quick and easy money, fast weight loss, or the next best thing for easily starting a business. In all of this, some of these things may be helpful, but they may not be helpful to us in our current situation. The only person who knows the information that we need to know is God, and the teacher He hires to teach us is the setback. The setback is on God's payroll, and it does its job wholeheartedly. Focus on the issue at hand and not everyone else attempting to teach or persuade you that their answer is better for your situation.

4. Ask questions. Learning comes by identifying and answering

questions. Questions help us wrap our minds around a given subject. They bring that subject into further clarity. The answers of life are found in questions, and we instinctively ask questions in times of setback, but seldom do we listen for a response. It's common to hear the question, "Why did this have to happen to me?" posed in times of setback. This isn't a bad question, but it's the action afterward that determines the meaningfulness and effectiveness of the question. What questions can be posed?—What can I learn from this situation? What is the reason for this happening at this moment and season of my life? What did I do right, and what have I done wrong? Whom can I turn to and learn from who has gone through the same thing? Where should I focus the majority of my attention?

5. Ask for the help of someone who understands the subject better than you do. This is self-explanatory. Seek the help of someone who understands a given area of life and has had a similar experience. This is the best person from whom to seek counsel. The added concern to this is that the person has to have acted properly and has to have come out of the setback with flying colors. Don't go to someone who has had a setback and handled it by cursing everyone out. This, of course, is a joke but the honest truth nonetheless. Gain wise counsel and not foolish counsel.

What not to do in setback's class. Here are the don'ts:

1. Don't listen inattentively. It's not wise to have our minds closed to teaching. We don't want to fall asleep on life and become bored. A closed mind doesn't grow, but ignored problems do.

2. Don't allow consensual distractions. Allowing distractions

to come uninhibitedly will only slow down the process of learning and permit the problem to resurface at a later date.

3. Don't have divided attention. Not everyone is the best to listen to and not everyone is a qualified teacher.

4. Don't refrain from asking questions. We can never sufficiently learn anything if we don't ask questions. When we do ask questions, we should seek a response.

5. Don't seek unwise counsel. We should not ask someone who is no more knowledgeable than we are or who offers unwise counsel for help.

Are you relieved now? Because that's all it takes to get the best grade you can, and it's also all it takes to face the tests over and over again. It's amazing how life offers us numerous chances to face, learn, and pass the tests that it offers. Seldom will we ever go to another level in life without first passing a test that would deem us qualified for that level. A stamp of approval coming from life issued by God is the highest honor we can have. The idea is to know and understand that just because we're sitting down doesn't mean that we can't learn.

It doesn't mean that we're not making progress. The place to learn is in the classroom, and then we go out into the field to do what we've just learned. So don't become discouraged if you're set down by life. It only wants to teach, and if we allow life to teach us, we're progressively moving forward. A setback is only designed to make us sit back,

> A setback is only designed to make us sit back, and sitting back is designed to help us look and observe the back end of what just happened to set us back.

and sitting back is designed to help us look and observe the back end of what just happened to set us back.

When I go to football games, I like to sit in the end zone seats. I love the end zone seats because they allow for a greater span of vision and also give a more realistic view of the on-field action. The best times are when they are just inside the twenty-yard line. It becomes close and personal. When they're on the other end, it's not as enjoyable, so sitting in the end zone has its ups and downs.

This situation is just like a setback. The up close and personal view, training, and revelation that we receive can sometimes be enjoyable because we are learning, but the downside to this is that sometimes it seems as if the action is leaving us as we sit, watch, and wait. Setbacks have their ups and downs, but if we can focus only on the ups, the downs won't mean much. This is an important note: just because the test is passed doesn't mean we won't have more of its kind. It only means that now we know how to deal with it constructively. A test can be administered at any time, so be ready.

Self-Motivation

Self-motivation is your ability to uplift yourself from the inside out by being knowledgeable about your abilities. Self-motivation is extremely important in the progressive movement in one's life. If people don't understand their abilities to become successful and move out of their old ways, they'll have trouble with progress. Trying to progress with minimal self-motivation is like trying to walk in quicksand. Every step we take toward progress will be slow and daunting—so much so that we may want to forget progress altogether.

Having self-motivation is less like running in quicksand and more like running on or in a Moonbounce. If you don't know what a Moonbounce is, it's the oversized, flat-surfaced balloon apparatus that kids jump on usually seen at carnivals. Self-motivation will send us afloat with each step. Self-motivation will keep us above any negative mind-sets, and most important, self-motivation will keep us energized, just like a kid on a Moonbounce.

Keep a Progress Log

Have you ever studied for the first time in months or years a picture of yourself that was taken years or months earlier? What was your reaction? Did you say, "Wow, I've changed a lot!" Some people may say they've gained weight, while some may say they've lost weight. Some notice they have gained an extra wrinkle, and some are reminded by a wild hairdo. However, most of us are surprised to see how much we've changed in this time. This is surprising because we're with ourselves every minute of the day, yet we fail to see the changes that our bodies undergo over time.

Sometimes, things are incredibly evident, and other times, things aren't so noticeable. We see ourselves so often that the little things are hard to track and follow. The same often goes for our progress. We want to keep track of our progress, because if we don't, we'll lose track of where we've improved. Buy a journal or a composition notebook and jot down weekly to monthly progress.

This practice is enjoyable because we can look back through our notes months later and be able to pinpoint major and minor events in our progress. We can even log our progress by digital voice recording. I'm more of a pen-and-paper person myself, but some may enjoy the digital recording. However it's done, it needs to happen. Tracking progress will also give way to self-critiquing and personal criticism.

If you find that you're not making progress, you can trace back through your recordings to see why. See what works and what doesn't. See what situations and circumstances send you back to your original mind-set. See what emotions arise when your old way of thinking emerges. You're something like a scientist observing yourself and learning about yourself.

Learning about ourselves is a new frontier for most of us. It's interesting how many of us barely know ourselves. We fail to realize why we do the things we do or why we're accustomed to certain patterns of thought. Have you noticed that your life is in patterns? Even your way of thinking is in patterns. This will be more evident to you as you begin a conscious process of progressing toward a successful state of mind.

Progress Tracking Tips

1. Write daily. Try your hardest to write each day about your actions in progress and actions that send you into regression.

2. Read your entries often, maybe not every day, but often enough that events of progress and events of regress are not easily forgotten.

3. Try to pinpoint feelings that sent you down the wrong road. Pinpoint feelings that you felt during the process and the feelings that you felt after the process.

4. Pinpoint thoughts and catalysts to thoughts that send you into a regressive state of mind. What do you see or hear or what do you remember that makes you decide to regress?

5. What time of the day do you feel most in tune with a progressive mind-set? And which time of the day do you feel the regressive mind-set in play?

6. All the same goes for a progressive mind-set also. Which thoughts send you into a conscious, progressive state of mind? What catalyst elements make for thoughts of progress?

Action Steps

1. Come to the realization that progress is a process that develops over time.

2. Use your time wisely by taking each day to improve your life or someone else's. Doing so allows progress to cling to you more.

3. Create momentum in your life by building on your successes.

4. Don't just move from a problem; act on the problem and come to a solution.

5. Realize solutions exist because problems exist. Problems are natural; solutions aren't.

6. Don't skip out on learning from your setbacks. Learn as much as you can from them and move on.

Station 11—
Being a Good Steward

"Being diligent to get is the easy part; being diligent to keep is what's difficult."

There are many things we come across that we have the opportunity to be good stewards over. Realizing the fact that nothing in our possession is ours but is loaned to us by God to manage will help us appreciate things more. Being a good steward starts at the level of appreciation and gratitude; those who are not good stewards are not appreciative of what they are given. We all fall victim to becoming unappreciative in one way or another. What are some things that we should be thankful for and become good stewards over? Time, possessions, resources, body, soul, and spirit are all good places to start.

Time

It's remarkable how everyone is allotted the same amount of time, and yet some people utilize their time more effectively than others. Just think of all the great thinkers, inventors, artists, musicians, preachers, and innovators; they all had the same amount of time in which to shape the world that we all have. How were they able to be so creative in the amount of time that they were given? They were good stewards over their time. I have so many thoughts in one day I have trouble tracing them all.

I constantly keep a pen by my side and a digital recorder to log all of my thoughts. I had and still have one problem if not checked that I must confess to. If I didn't plan my day and stick to the schedule, I would be everywhere and wouldn't get anything done. My mind is racing every minute of the day, and when I get in front of books, it's even worse. I could begin one thing, and something else would attract my attention, and then I'd be off to that.

On and on it goes until I find myself doing nothing. In these moments of time, I wasn't being a good steward. Even though I was reading and working, I wasn't being a good steward because I knew how I functioned and still didn't do anything to resolve the issue. It's a lesson that I had to learn since no one can do anything worthwhile when his or her focus is everywhere. Time is one of our most precious commodities, and it's the easiest to let slip from our hands.

No one can ever get a firm grasp on time, but we can all learn how to work with time. Time is like a mail carrier; both the carrier and time deliver in all sorts of conditions. The motto is "through hail, sleet, and snow." Time is willing to help us if we are willing to help ourselves. Time will say, "Okay, I'll work with you, but only if you're willing to work with me, because I'm busy."

Possessions

We often crave more than we need. We are never satisfied with what we have and are always coming up with excuses for why we should get what we want. The question we should ask ourselves is: "Am I a good steward over the little that I do have?" Now, you may be saying, "Of course I am. I keep all of my things in excellent condition," but being a good steward doesn't end there. Being a good steward is also being thankful and content with the things you have.

Contentment is a big, nasty word that no one really likes. What we have to understand is that contentment isn't a bad thing. Mastering the art of being content is a way to keep us sane and keep us from throwing our lives away trying to live something that is far from us. Not everyone is going to be a millionaire, but all of us have the ability to live comfortably and to give to others in need and lack. We have to understand that contentment is an outward focus.

When we look at what we have, we should be calmly pleased with felicity. We should be grateful and understand that there are millions of people around the world who can't buy something as simple as a sandwich. The only object we should show discontent toward is our inner being. Discontent is an inner focus, meaning that we should always strive for more internally. We should be striving and craving for more knowledge, wisdom, and understanding; this form of discontent is acceptable.

When the two are reversed what we have then is a person who is content internally and discontent externally. Their focus is all wrong. This is the mind-set of most people. These individuals are more apt to strive for outer things than they are for inner things. They are, in essence, average and mediocre individuals with issues of coveting and lusting for possessions. If we focus on being content outwardly or externally and on being discontent inwardly and internally, we'll balance the wheel of life that spins in us all.

If we find ourselves being discontent on the inside, what we're essentially doing is creating within ourselves more of the things that draw the outward things, so automatically, as we work on the inner self, the less significant outer things will crown our lives, honoring good stewardship. People try to draw material things to themselves by artifice in the forms of crime and avarice, but no one can trick nature for long; eventually, nature will correct the wrongs. Therefore, it's wise not to start down this path but to do the necessary things to build the inner person. As I like to say, "Don't put success on credit. Work hard now, and save up the wisdom you'll need to pay full price for true and good success."

> As I like to say, "Don't put success on credit. Work hard now, and save up the wisdom you'll need to pay full price for true and good success."

What are we doing with the things we do have? Are we utilizing them sufficiently, or are we squandering them on ourselves? When asking God for anything, we can't ask Him with the intention of using it for our own selfish pleasures. Doing so will be like talking into the air; therefore, those things in our possession aren't meant for our use only but also to help others. This is a tough one, I know, but it's true.

We get satisfaction out of helping others, but we can't help someone with something that we don't have. As I mentioned earlier, I also had to transform my way of thinking concerning this subject, because I always believed that the next person wasn't going to take care of my possessions as I took care of them. In one instance, someone borrowed something of mine without returning it, and I was vehemently concerned about the transgression, but as the Bible denotes in Proverbs, the book of wisdom, "A man's wisdom gives him patience; it is to his glory to overlook an offense."[8] So just like in this example, sometimes, occurrences like this will happen, but it is to our glory to still lend a helping hand in spite of them and again show mercy by overlooking an offense against us.

This is one of the reasons that most people refuse to share their possessions. Let it be noted, however, that it's an offense if we don't lend our possessions but instead say to a person that we don't have something when we do. This is counted against us. So being a good steward also means sharing with others. Even if its knowledge about something, don't be so prideful and arrogant as not to help someone else who is in need of the information that you have.

However, be wise and judge carefully. I wouldn't recommend allowing just anyone to borrow your car even if the person is family. You must use discretion. It wouldn't hurt to give that person a ride if need be. But once again, use sagacity. Never pick up a complete stranger. Plus, you'll know the difference between a person who is in need and a person who wants to covet your possessions. Overall, the idea is to help others with what you have.

Resources

How is it possible to be a good steward over resources? What are some resources that we have at our use? Money, knowledge, friendships, education, experiences, and associations, among others. Remember, being good stewards means being people who put their possessions to good use. Now, to this statement, we will add this stipulation to good stewardship: not only should we put them to good use, but if they can be multiplied, they should be multiplied.

Money is one thing that can be multiplied by savings and investments. Money is also something that can play a huge factor in how we live our lives and who we call lord—being the one who has power, authority, and influence over us. Sometimes, we allow money to be our lord—this isn't being a good steward. Money isn't meant to rule over us even though money has unmistakable influence. The influence of money should be used for good and not evil.

Gifts and talents are other possessions that can be multiplied. All gifts and talents given to us should be nursed and built upon. All gifts and talents in our possession were given to us for a purpose; it's best to make the best use of them. Mold and craft these gifts and talents into skills. When we develop our gifts and talents into skills, we set ourselves apart from those who only rely on their raw talents and abilities. This is what sets professionals apart from amateurs.

Body

There is one thing that we are very conscious of, and that is a healthy body. So many ailments and diseases can attack people who aren't good stewards over their bodies. We need regular exercise and proper diets to keep us in good health. Ask yourself, "Am I showing God gratitude by keeping this temple healthy? Am I really thankful that I have this body?" It's good to be thankful even in this instance because a lot of people weren't born with the full use of their bodies.

They were never given the chance to be able to appreciate the benefits of taking care of their bodies to the extent that healthy, fully functioning people can. Our health is one of the most important things that we have. If we don't have our health, how will we be able to mange our daily lives and enjoy the people in them? It's not fun trying to enjoy family or friends while in discomfort and pain.

Soul

The soul is the creativity compartment of a human being. From the soul, creativity is conceived. Being a good steward over the soul entails being cognizant of that to which we lend our minds, ears, and eyes. Our soul is fed by way of these gates. Even to some extent, touch, feeling, and smell are also gateways to the soul.

Being extra careful not to overindulge ourselves with the wrong forms of inspiration is important. Our souls are diluted in this day. It's evident that not many people would go and see a movie in which animals were being tortured, and rightly so; animal cruelty is an atrocity. Not many people would go see entertainment of something of this sort, but how many of us would go and see a movie about helpless people being tortured and call it entertainment? Our souls have been polluted with all sorts of violence and degradations of human life, so that we have become extremely calloused.

Our soul was given to us so that we could express love and compassion for our fellow humans. It was given to us so that we could express ourselves in ways that others could also enjoy. The soul is the area in which we connect with people and things. We have to take the steps to beautify our souls again. We have to deprogram ourselves from the callousness and disregard of compassion for human life. Whatever is happening in our souls is happening in our lives, because the soul is the tool or unit of expression.

Spirit

The spirit is the part of the human being that is everlasting. The spirit cannot perish, so it perpetuates for eternity. The spirit is one of the units that make up the being of a person; the function of the sprit is to connect us with God. The spirit of man and woman is sustained by spiritual things, so read the Bible. A lack of scripture in our lives is a lack of stewardship for our spirits.

Action Steps

1. Become grateful for all the good things in your life, even down to the smallest thing.
2. Be aware that being a good steward over time is a necessity. Time is something that we can never get back.
3. Possessions are given to us by God even if it feels like we acquired them on our own. This is His common grace. Therefore, share with others and improve their lives.
4. Multiply what you can, and never sit on your talents and gifts. They will only improve when used.

5. Exercise regularly. There are many books and magazines that will specify what it takes to live a physically healthy life.

6. Protect your soul by protecting your ears and your eyes. Feed your soul with wholesome material.

Station 12—Living

"The great paradox about life is that life comes from death. What has to die in you in order that you may have life?"

To live or not to live, that is the question. To live is the question. The response is, "Am I living?" As we've gone through preparation for success, determination, progress, being a good steward, and now living, we see that each chapter is an incremental step to the next. Preparation is the first step to living; therefore, preparation is a precondition to living a full life.

Once preparation begins, there must be determination and persistence to continue with the process. No time is wasted because you have a clear-cut goal prescribed to the conditions you would like to meet. You've set your mind and have decided to push through with your plans; therefore, progress will ensue. If you desire success and a goal-specific mind-set, progress will be evident. Progress presents new and better situations, and with new situations comes more responsibility and a greater level of stewardship.

The quality of stewardship, however, doesn't start after progress but begins before your current aim of progress. Being a good steward brings more progress as a result. This all leads up to the final thing to do, and that is to live. To live means to carry joy and happiness in your daily walk. It means to be self-aware and be alert to yourself and your environment. It means that we should have a level of pride and respect for things in our possession, and it means to live a righteous life before God.

The famous, wealthy, and wise King Solomon summed up the meaning of life in a few simple points. First and foremost, the duty of all mankind is to serve God wholeheartedly. Second, you should love your family (which includes *all* people), and last, you should work assiduously so that you may be able to be a blessing to others—in all of this, you are living a full life. This is coming from a man who wrote three thousand wise sayings; he sums up life in only three points. The world can be complex, but life generally isn't as difficult as we choose to make it. Yet, we struggle with conjoining these points.

Some choose to say that there is no God; some dislike the family they were given, and then others struggle with slothfulness. What more would we need if we had these three points fulfilled? We have communion with the God who created us. We love our families; we have enough money to take care of them, live a modest life, and have the ability to provide for others' needs. Now combine these three points and imagine how that may be. Sounds like a utopia? Sounds inconceivable? Well, it isn't.

Joy

There is much joy to experience in this world, but it's hard to come by when stress and pain are crippling the mind. If joy was the sun, then circumstances and problems would be dark rain clouds that block the sun's light. One of the reasons we have trouble escaping this cloud is that we have the proclivity to be too concerned about

> We are the initiators of our joy.

our own lives. Once we learn that doing for others is the beginning of joy, we'll experience it more often. We are the initiators of our joy. We are responsible for ourselves, either in having joy or in having sorrow.

So then, what's the problem? Why are so many us joy deficient? I believe sometimes the problem lies in the false assumption that giving of ourselves to others will leave us with less. The famous question is: "Well, what about me?" Life does an incredible job of supporting the *correct* system.

That system entails giving one another support and supplying the needs of those around us; by doing so, miraculously, we get back more than we gave. How does this happen? To be honest, I don't know; I don't have an intelligent enough answer. It's just the way God made things; we are to give support to one another and perpetuate life. But as we can see, we humans like to take more than we give, and our world is seeing and feeling the effects.

Instead of perpetuating life by support and giving, we perpetuate death by undermining and taking. I have a friend who has a heart for the well-being of people. Identifying the fact that many people in the inner cities of America are the ones who need the most help, he set up a parachurch to help feed and improve the lives of these people. He has a tremendous heart for others, and as we've learned, a heart is a true belief. He truly believes that these people can improve their lives, but only if someone who is capable will help.

Resources and support come from the most unlikely places, and he has much joy in his heart. His compassion for people is what drives him to help them, and his passion to serve God is what sustains him. As I like to say, "Passion is for us; compassion is for others." We should always have passion burning inside of us to keep us going, but we should never have sympathy for ourselves. Sympathy is for others, especially those who are less fortunate than we are.

As an analogy, look at the Dead Sea; it allows water to flow in but doesn't allow water to flow out, so the Dead Sea is stagnating. Another word for stagnant is *dead*, hence the name, the Dead Sea. When we allow our lives to become stagnant only allowing ourselves to receive, we become like the Dead Sea, which is hazardous. It's hazardous to ourselves and to the people around us. I cannot stress the importance of helping out our fellow human beings and showing compassion to those people enough. "These things have I spoken unto you, that my joy might remain in you, and that your joy might be full. This is my commandment, that ye love one another, as I have loved you."[9]

Happiness

Happiness is the fruit of joy. Happiness is a result of being content outwardly and inwardly discontent. It is the fruit of giving of ourselves to help others. It is the fruit of having fun with family and friends, and the laughter that tickles our belly.If joy was the sun, happiness would be the exhilaration and excitement we have while playing at the beach and enjoying the sun.

Happiness is secondary and comes after primary needs are met. Most people try to make happiness primary while the things that bring happiness are deemed unimportant. Happiness isn't found in money and possessions; money and possessions only bring limited, temporary happiness. However, money is one of the subcategories that bring forth happiness. It should be noted that the idea of having money for the sake of having it isn't what brings happiness.

It's what we constructively do with money in helping others that brings happiness. There was a young man long ago who was very wealthy. There was also a very popular teacher who was transcending the times. This teacher spoke the truth forcefully with vehement desire, and some were intrigued, like this young man. One day, the young man approached this teacher and inquired of him, "What must I do to come into perpetual life?"

The teacher replied, "Have you kept your character intact? Have you obeyed the simplest of principles that would lead a person to have a blameless and successful life?"

And the young man answered, "Yes, sir, I have. I have honored all of these things."

The teacher peered at the young man as he responded, "You lack one thing. Sell everything you have and give to the poor, and you will have treasure in an immense and unyielding kingdom."

After this, the wealthy young man became very sad, and he walked away, head down and dejected.[10] Some people may think it was harsh to say to the young man, "Sell everything you have," but the principle of this story can be seen in a few points:

Having money and possessions can play a big part in your happiness, but if these possessions are hoarded, what good will they do to bring happiness? All who have stingily kept their possessions to themselves will only walk away sad like the young man. Money and possessions can either bring happiness or sadness.

The teacher was showing the young man where his heart was. No matter how tightly we walk the rope, if others are not included in our endeavors, we are only blowing our efforts into the wind.

Outwardly, this young man was alive, but inwardly, he was dead. He was stagnant and deficient of the correct system. So no new thing could flow through him, like the possessions of the kingdom of which the teacher spoke.

Side Note: Giving from an ungrateful heart is just as bad as not giving at all. It doesn't specifically say this in this particular story, but the attitude of the young man would suggest that he would reluctantly give his possessions just to come into possession of eternal life, and if this is the case, he might as well keep his possessions.

I understand that I've been ranting and raving about giving, but giving is the only way to receive happiness. In order to be happy with a spouse, close friend, family member, or co-worker, we must make some sacrifices. We must give of ourselves if we want to receive the same love and affection. The selfish person who is snobby has few friends. Who wants to be around someone who only takes? No one does! This is why giving is the primary cause of happiness. Giving equals others; others equal joy; and joy equates to happiness.

Self-Awareness

To live a full life, we must become self-aware. One of the first steps to success is having our awareness centered on the truth about ourselves. Self-awareness is as simple as it sounds; it's how aware we are of ourselves. Do we really know ourselves as well as we would like to think? We have to be cognizant of our own habits of thought, our strengths and weaknesses, and how we relate to people or the world around us, and identify the things about ourselves we are willing to c h a n g e .

Self-awareness comes before self-esteem in that we have to be sure of ourselves before we can esteem ourselves. Those people who are sure of themselves have high self-esteem; they are aware of their habits of thought, their strengths, and their weaknesses.

> Self-awareness comes before self-esteem in that we have to be sure of ourselves before we can esteem ourselves.

They know what makes them, them. How can people live a complete life when they don't fully understand themselves? They don't understand the way in which they think or why they like what they like and dislike what they dislike. That can be a confusing world.

Knowing ourselves will help us in every area of our lives, especially in the workforce. When we can discover what really drives us, it gives us the incentive to work with all of our might toward whatever we put our hands to. For example, I grew up unaware of why I disliked the way that some people thought and went about their lives. It irritated me for so long that I began to be unsure of myself. I began to have thoughts that maybe I was a Goody Two-shoes, as the saying goes, or I wasn't as cool as the rest of the kids.

This wasn't the case at all. God had given me the ability to see the world differently. The traps that most adolescents fall into and have trouble finding their way out of, God colored in bright reds and yellows for me. Is this something to brag about? Of course not, but what God has done is given me experiences so that I may teach others. I've always been a strong proponent of renewing the mind for the better.

I knew that the only way to be transformed was by the renewing of the mind. Therefore, what I do now I love. I've placed my hand to the plow, and I'm not looking back. I've found enjoyable work for my hands to do, and I do it with all of my might. This is because I became aware of myself. I became aware of what I'm here to accomplish.

I'm now aware that I wasn't weird but just thought differently from the rest. I know my strengths, the things that I gain strength and vigor in doing, and my weaknesses, the things that I find dread in doing. The best thing about being self-aware is that now I can pour all of my energy into doing the things that make me stronger and work at perfecting those things. Now I can live and have the full life that God promised me, and this is only because I became self-aware. It's amazing how much we try to hide ourselves from ourselves.

Have you ever come into contact with people who will not admit that they have a problem even though it's as clear as the blue sky? *Denial* is the proper term here. They deny that they have any problems at all.

These people are choosing to be unaware of themselves, and this is bad for them. Why? Because they're never going to open up to see what good things they have on the inside of themselves.

Covering up one thing leads to the covering up of more things, even the good things. It's kind of like having an extremely junky closet; if you open it, everything in it will fall out, but amongst the mess hangs a beautiful garment. There may be good things hanging up on the inside of us, but if we are afraid to open up based on the junk, the good things will go undiscovered and untapped. We have to take responsibility for the junk we have in our closets and clean them out.

Tips to becoming self-aware:

Take an inventory of your likes and dislikes and state why you like/dislike them.

See where you stand with family and friends. How are you perceived by the ones close to you?

How do you relate to the world?

Pay attention to how you *react* to certain situations and circumstances. Be honest when you notice your tendencies.

Pride

In some instances, pride is a horrible thing. Pride in the form of stubbornness is a horrid trait to have, but pride in the sense of gaining satisfaction from a job well done is necessary. There is nothing like the feeling of accomplishing a goal that has taken time and effort to complete. Whenever my father works on a project, he has a certain level of pride connected to his work. He once told me a story about working with someone who thought it was okay to overlook a mistake because no one would see.

My dad, being the honest person he is, corrected the gentleman by saying that he didn't do anything halfheartedly and knowing that he saw it and God saw it was enough to know that covering it up was wrong.

Because he has this level of pride in his work, he has people calling him often wanting something of theirs fixed or built. They understand that he has pride in what he does. They understand that he operates in honesty and what he builds will have a hard time falling.

My mother is a homemaker. She has pride in the way she takes care of my father. Every morning, she is up early with him as she sees him off to work and prepares a meal before he comes home. This may seem old-fashioned, but it may be a testament to their happily lived thirty-seven plus years of marriage to date. My siblings and I never wanted for anything because my mother and father made sure we had what we needed. They took pride in how they raised us.

We hear the word *pride* in school fight songs and chants. We talk about school spirit as a tradition. In the month of March, we can turn to a basketball game and see the school spirit and pride that the students have for their team. Ranting and raving, they show how dedicated they are, sometimes sleeping out in the rain just to get a ticket for the game. That's dedication; that's pride. How is pride developed?

It's developed by having an appreciation for something and taking responsibility for it. It's also created by having a certain level of dedication to wanting the best, striving for the best, and giving your best. Pride is also built by having a sense of ownership. Anyone who owns anything thinks differently toward it. First-time homeowners are thrilled to be able to call their house home.

They take care of the house and the yard. They are what they call "proud homeowners." A sense of ownership will always heighten the level of pride in a person, because ownership heightens responsibility, appreciation (in some regards), and dedication. If there isn't anything that you can say you're proud of, you're not fully living. At a sports event, when all of the students are standing on their feet and yelling at the tops of their lungs, we can see that they all come alive. Their senses are heightened, and they're ready to explode in an uproar of praise for good play. They're alive!

Pride doesn't just come; pride develops through building on ownership, dedication, appreciation, and responsibility. If you lack pride in something, it may be because you lack a certain level of integrity that would allow for a sense of wanting to do things the right way. It may be because there is a lack of responsibility or connection. It may be because there is a lack of dedication. I believe this is the most common reason to have a deficiency in pride: a lack of dedication.

One thing to be aware of is the fine line between good pride and bad pride. Good pride is built on the characteristics mentioned above; bad pride is pride that takes one from having joy to having a keen sense of awful stubbornness. This form of pride is one step before ruin. This pride is horrid in that to these people, good sportsmanship is only a term found in the dictionary that doesn't apply to them. For the homeowners, being good sportsmen is being people who take care of their home but not so that they can put other homes to shame.

You know the guy who only plants grass seed and mows his lawn so that he can make his neighbor's lawn look like the Sahara Desert? In this case, the man should care for his lawn to keep his house up, not to embarrass someone else. Whenever the aim or objective of our pride is to humiliate someone else, we have overstepped our boundaries. Our pride should be situated in such a way that our labor brings joy to ourselves as well as others; it should never be used to demean anyone.

Righteousness

Our world has fallen into decay and decadence. The minds of people have descended into a dark abyss of immorality and indecency. Nothing seems to be sacred anymore. Everything is up to relative terms or means. We make our own beliefs; we make our own truths and objectivity.

The world is becoming a scary place in which to live, but

nevertheless, we must live. If nature could have its way, it wouldn't believe in relativity; it would believe and live by objectivity, as it does. All of God's creations, besides the human race, abide by the same set of rules and laws they were subjected to from the beginning, and it seems to be fairing out well for them. Their objective life has brought much abundance for them, and if it wasn't for humans destroying their way of life (ecosystem), they would continue to flourish and live for hundreds and thousands of years more. This isn't an attempt to demean the human race, but it is an attempt to show that as intelligent as humans are, we can get in our own way sometimes.

What I'm referring to here is the natural principles set into place that would ensure us abundance and success; righteousness is one of those principles, not simply from a religious standpoint but from that of the collective whole of all mankind. What truth do we objectively live our lives by? Do we believe life happened by chance? If we believe that life happened by chance, there is no need to live righteously. Nothing would really matter.

Some people would say we decide what is meaningful in life. If this is true, then why decide to live in right standing? To live in right standing would mean that there is an original truth to live by. If there is no original truth to judge by, what then would be injustice or wrongdoing? Who could decide based on a world built by chance?

I believe one of the reasons the United States Constitution has stood as one of the world's greatest documents is because it is based on unquestionable, undeniable truth, which would then mean nothing has happened by chance but by purpose. Instead of living with purpose, we try to live on purpose. The difference is when people try to live on purpose, they purposely buy and surround themselves with the things that they believe will create a

> Instead of living with purpose, we try to live on purpose.

purposeful life for them—a nice car, nice clothes, a nice house, and well-known friends. A purposeful life can only be lived when we live with purpose.

As we live with purpose, our life is defined for us, and we don't have to try to live on purpose. Our lives are purposeful and intended by a higher power who knew good and well what they were doing in creating us. If we were made in the likeness of an objective God, then we too should strive to live objectively. Righteously, we're to see the injustices in the world and do what is in our power to avert them. Begin today to live with purpose and right the wrongs and injustices that are rampant in our world.

Bringing Life to Visions, Dreams, and Goals

The female race has the extraordinary task of perpetuating life. Through the female is life continued and nurtured. What an amazing ability! All people walking on the face of this earth have had a mother who carried them roughly nine months and then birthed them. Why is this important to us? If we want our visions, dreams, or goals to grow into maturity, we will need to mentally adopt the characteristics representative of the female race. What are some of these characteristics? They are being nurturers, being intuitive, being emotionally driven, being connectors (connecting one event to another), being comforters, being bearers of life, and being compassionate.

Being Nurturers

In the context of adopting the characteristics of a nurturer, what we're doing is developing the know-how that involves the process of taking care of our aspirations (visions, dreams, and goals). By becoming nurturers, we develop the mind-set and right attitude that will assist us in encouraging our aspirations to grow and flourish. We extend a helping hand with tender care and protection all the while fending for our aspirations so they have the right to live. We have to be careful never to push our visions, dreams, and goals past the competence of their current level of maturity. Many times, people have taken their visions, dreams, and goals and have pushed them out of the nest too soon, and since the wings were still weak, they fell to the ground. Being a nurturer calls for an observant attitude, looking over and after the aspiration until it can fend for itself in spite of ridicule and doubters who would try to cripple its growth.

Being Intuitive

There is one thing that all mothers seem confident in knowing and that is the sound of their child's cry. I've seen mothers on the playground who instinctively knew the sound of their child's voice over the multitude of voices typical at a park or playground. These mothers are in tune with their children. Through communion with their children, they have built a certain decisive and appropriate "knowing." This is only built through having a strong connection.

Knowing directly and instinctively about the state of a vision, dream, or goal is a trait best suited for those who have a deep commitment to it. Our goals and desires speak to us. They let us know what's going on, and if we're truly committed, we'll know exactly what they are saying. Is it time to add? Is it time to grow? Is it time to move on, to simplify, to push harder, slow down, calm down, or feed its hunger? It'll speak its desire or need to us; our only job is to listen when it does.

Being Emotionally Driven

God has given women the ability to be emotionally driven. This was by no means given by chance but so that women could be excellent motivators. Women are able to motivate and persuade even when the motivation is done in a way that is perverted to God's will. If the use of her emotions is self-centered and manipulative, this is a perversion, but

Charles T. Robinson Jr.

effective nonetheless. This capacity to get things done and attain results is a must and a needed trait for anyone with a lofty goal. Anyone with a winning attitude is emotionally driven. Those who have won anything remember how good it felt to win; therefore, winning is derived from feeling, emotion, and attitude.

If we want to be a winner in the race of getting our desires across the finish line, we have to be emotionally driven with a winner's attitude. Now this isn't loose or out-of-control emotion but centered and concentrated emotion. Take note, emotion isn't all that's needed to get a vision on its feet, because there is a certain level of logic and application. But firm, definite, and concentrated emotion, which consists of passion, dedication, perseverance, determination, big-picture thinking, love, hope, and compassion, are big and helpful proponents. If we are driven by these things, we will surely see ourselves stepping over the finish line alongside our goals. This is how we persuade ourselves and motivate ourselves to attain results and get things done.

Being Connectors

Women, by nature, are connectors. They have the tendency to relate one life circumstance to another. Everything is connected in an interconnecting web. For this reason, it's good for anyone to have the connector quality concerning visions, dreams, and goals. Opportunity is all around us. Most thoughts come in a single form, but because of their attentiveness to opportunity, some people are able to combine indirect or unrelated qualities concerning those thoughts and are able to enhance them. Some people call this creativity.

In this form of thinking, we are allowing our dreams to become social. What I mean by social is we are not allowing our dreams to be cut off from gaining valuable wisdom and forming relationships that can help push them along. No one who is a recluse can ever be fully successful because no one person has all the answers. If your dream

176

could talk literally, it would have many associates to glean from; at least this is how it should be. We must learn to be connectors.

Being Comforters

We've all done it; through the midnight hour, we have awoken and cried aloud for someone to come and comfort us, preferably with a hot bottle of milk. Who walks into the room? Either Mommy or Daddy, it doesn't matter; all we wanted was comfort. The same is true when running the obstacle course of life. We'll have our ups and downs. We'll have to climb and dive. We'll have to walk and crawl. We'll have to dodge doubters and embrace criticism, and we'll have to find comfort from all the pains and struggles. I can only imagine what it's like for an infant. Waking up in the middle of the night wondering, *Where is everyone?* Just like that infant, many adults wake up to see another day and another reason to need comfort, because there is no one around to help them toward their goals. Some do, but many don't, and just like the parents throw a warm comforter across their children's bodies to keep them warm, adults need the same, metaphorically. We develop this comfort, and we relieve ourselves of grief and anxiety by reminding ourselves that no one can stop us but us.

Along with this is knowing that God has given us the right not to worry or be anxious about anything but to cast all cares upon Him. Comfort is found in promises that can't be broken and faith. Even I have had to encourage and comfort myself while penning this book by reminding myself of my promises and the faith that I have in my Lord. Everyone has those days of discomfort, grief, and anxiety, wondering if they are worthy even to consider chasing after their vision; the answer is always a resounding yes. Nothing can stop a flower from growing if it goes untouched. In the event of something blocking its sunlight, it will lean into the direction of the most sunlight so that it can continue to grow. This is true for us also; no one can stop us but us, and when there is hindrance to our growth, we should just lean to find the light.

Being a Bearer of Life

Do you bear life in your speech? Take a quick inventory of your habits of speech. What does it consist of? Is there any inkling of "I can't" or "I'm not good enough"? What about "I'm not smart enough"?

Life can only perpetuate where there is life. If there isn't any life in our speech, then there cannot be life in our dreams. Out of the abundance of the heart, the mouth speaks. If we want our goals to reach maturity, we must be cognizant of our speech, which ultimately comes from what we believe. What are we saying and believing about ourselves?

What are we saying and believing about others? Everything adds up in our quest for success. We want the environment of our vision, dream, or goal to be positive so that it may grow. We don't want it around any pollution. Bear life in your speech, and you will bear life in your dreams.

Being Compassionate

Compassion is nothing more than passion that is compressed—compressed passion. Passion is usually thought of as intense emotion, while compassion is this in a condensed and controlled state. The technical description for it is sympathy for the suffering of others and a desire to help. In the case of Jesus, as He showed His compassion for the people, He was intensely motivated and moved to help those with a burning desire and passion. In our visions, dreams, and goals, the best way to see them through to completion is to set a goal that will help others.

Whether it's family, friends, or strangers, we must develop a sense of compassion. For example, even if the goal that we're trying to obtain is that of personal health, keeping ourselves healthy is not just for us but for our families also. We want to help ourselves live longer so that we can be around longer for our families. Compassion will move us to do things that we normally wouldn't do, like give a kidney to a dying person or give bone marrow. Compassion is a motivator, and it will move us. If our aspiration consists of helping people, then the trait of compassion will move us to keep going and not to quit. Not everyone's goals will be as easy to connect to others. This doesn't necessarily mean that they're wrong, but each of us should have a goal that is directly related to someone other than ourselves. We may reap the benefits, but we can tie the desire to someone else.

Action Steps

1. Begin to do more for others, whether it's holding the door for the next person or volunteering at a homeless shelter.
2. Realize that joy starts with serving and giving to others.
3. Find a reason to be happy. If you have your health or if you have somewhere to call home, you should be happy.
4. Develop a sense of ownership for things that you otherwise wouldn't. Take on the responsibility.
5. Eagerly develop and build the character that is necessary for the growth of your aspirations.

To contact this author

personaltrainerforthemind@hotmail.com

or to visit blog

www.personaltrainerforthemind.com

(Endnotes)

Station 1—The Warm-Up: Take a Lap with Me

[1]*Webster's New Explorer Dictionary and Thesaurus*, New ed. (Springfield: Federal Street Press, 2005), s.v. "create."

[2]Ibid., s.v. "thinking."

[3]Phil. 4:8, NIV.

[4]John Maxwell, *Thinking For A Change: 11 Ways Highly Successful People Approach Life and Work* (New York: Warner Books Inc, 2003), 183.

Station 2—Stretching the Mind: Full Range of (E)motion

[1] Romans 1:20, AMP.

[2] Hosea 4:6, NIV.

[3]*Webster's New Explorer*, s.v. "passion."

[4]Matthew 21:12-13, AMP.

Station 4—Losing Weight: Step on My Mental Scale

[1]*Webster's New Explorer*, s.v. "discouragement."

[2] Matthew 7:12, AMP.

Station 6—Mental Endurance: Breathe Inspiration to Sustain Life and Health

[1]*Webster's New Explorer*, s.v. "inspiration."

Station 7—Arriving at Your Destination

[1]Proverbs 18:16, KJV.

Station 8—Preparation for Success

[1]Matthew 25:1–13, NIV.

Station 9—Determination and Persistence

[1]*Webster's New Explorer*, s.v. "deter."
[2]*Webster's New Explorer*, s.v. "terminate."

Station 11—Being a Good Steward

[1]Proverbs 19:11, NIV.

Station 12—Live

[1]John 15:11–12, KJV.
[2] Luke 18:18–23, NIV.